Contents

Domestic violence:

a health care issue?

British Medical Association

June 1998

Domestic violence: a health care issue?

A publication from the British Medical Association Science Department and the Board of Science and Education

Chairman, Board of Science and Education:	Professor Jack Howell
Head, Professional Resources and Research Group:	Professor Vivienne Nathanson
Editor:	Dr David R Morgan
Contributing Authors:	Lisa Davies Dr Lorraine Radford[1] Dr Jo Richardson[2]
Editorial Secretariat:	Dawn Whyndham
Indexer:	Richard Jones
Design:	Hilary Glanville

British Library Cataloguing in Publication Data. A catalogue record for this book is available from the British Library.

ISBN 0 7279 1370 0

First published in 1998 by the British Medical Association, Tavistock Square, London, WC1H 9JP
Printed by: The Chameleon Press, London.

Cover Photograph:	Richard Schneider, Image Bank Photo Library

---

1.   Senior Lecturer in Social Policy. Roehampton Institute, London.
2.   General Practitioner, East London. Research Fellow, Department of General Practice and Primary Care, St Bartholomew's, London and the Royal London School of Medicine and Dentistry, Queen Mary and Westfield College, London.

1 Introduction

The British Medical Association (BMA) is the professional organisation representing all doctors in the UK. It was established in 1832 to *promote the medical and allied sciences, and to maintain the honour of the profession.* The Board of Science and Education, a standing committee of the Association, supports this aim by acting as an interface between the profession, the government and the public, and by undertaking research studies on behalf of the BMA. Through the publication of policy statements, the Board of Science and Education has led the debate on key public health and professional issues.

The overriding objective of the Board is to contribute to the development of better public health policies that affect the community, the state and the medical profession. In order to do this, investigations are carried out by the Board to examine the impact of various policies and activities on the public health. The Board appoints working parties and steering groups, combining medical and other specialist expertise to carry out research on a variety of important issues. The Board has published a large number of reports over recent years reflecting current concerns in the public health arena such as complementary medicine, health inequalities, transport policy and environmental issues and the misuse of drugs.

The Board also has responsibility for educational initiatives. Many of the reports published through the Board are used in medical education programmes, additionally the Board's publications have been used in schools and higher education. The Board not only develops such educational materials but also has an interest in educational policy.

Domestic violence and the BMA

At the BMA's 1996 Annual Representative Meeting (ARM) it was resolved that *the Board of Science and Education should examine the long term health implications of domestic violence.* Following consideration of the resolution, the Board agreed that the remit of the resolution should concentrate on all types of abuse between sexual partners and would not consider other aspects of family violence, including child abuse which is covered by the work of another BMA working party on child health. However, it was emphasised that the effects of this violence would have wider consequences beyond the individual involved and could relate to children and other relatives. Therefore the impact of domestic violence on children is discussed in some detail in Chapter Four.

As domestic violence has received little attention in health care settings in the UK until fairly recently, the Board of Science and Education agreed that this study should consider domestic violence as a health care issue. This present report is therefore intended to be a comprehensive but accessible discussion document, to raise awareness of the nature and prevalence of domestic violence and to discuss the role of health care workers in identifying the problem and to devise strategies to help to manage and reduce the problem. Chapter Six concentrates in detail on the role of general practice, but it is not intended to cover such detail for every specialty as this issue has been addressed by some of the Royal Colleges; in particular an excellent report, *Violence Against Women*, has been produced by the Royal College of Obstetricians and Gynaecologists.[1]

Domestic violence as a health issue

The impact which domestic violence has will vary from person to person, but there is growing evidence to confirm that it does have serious and long lasting consequences on the health and well being of the individual.

In 1996, the World Medical Association issued a declaration on family violence, which included domestic violence. They recommended that national medical associations should encourage and facilitate research to understand the prevalence, risk factors, outcomes, and optimal care for those who have experienced family violence. They also state that doctors have an important role to play in the prevention and treatment of family violence.[2]

In the Annual Report of the Chief Medical Officer for England and Wales *On the State of the Public Health 1996,* domestic violence has been highlighted as a special area for consideration during 1998. The report states that domestic violence has considerable implications for the NHS — particularly in accident and emergency departments, primary care and in specialist settings such as maternity services and child and adolescent mental health services.[3]

We regret that no reference to domestic violence is made in the recent Government publications: *The White Paper: the Future of the NHS*[4] and the Green Paper *Our Healthier Nation,*[5] although we applaud the reference to it in the Scottish Green Paper, *Working Together for a Healthier Scotland.*[6] Domestic violence is a national problem and a national framework is required to ensure a basic standard of care for all.

The Primary Care Groups and the Health Improvement Programmes suggested by the recent White and Green Papers for England and Wales and Scotland[7,8,9,10] may provide more opportunity for a policy on management referral for inter-agency co-ordination initiatives. There is scope for the NHS to make greater strides in the development of policy and practice in relation to patients who experience domestic violence, but as yet there is no firm policy in this area.

It is therefore intended that this timely BMA report on domestic violence should lead the way in encouraging the medical profession to raise their awareness of the problem, and to develop strategies to identify and reduce the health implications caused by this major public health problem.

As little is known about the long term health implications connected with domestic violence further research is needed. The Board therefore recommended to the Trustees that research funds of £17,000 from the BMA Joan Dawkins Trust Fund should be allocated to a project to research the physical, psychological and social health implications of domestic violence and this will commence in 1998.

Board of Science and Education

This report was prepared under the auspices of the Board of Science and Education of the BMA. The members of the Board were:

Acknowledgements

The Association is grateful for the specialist help provided by the BMA Committees and many outside experts and organisations and would particularly like to thank Dr Iona Heath, General Practitioner, Kentish Town, North London and Dr Gillian Mezey, Senior Lecturer and Consultant, Forensic Psychiatry, St George's Hospital Medical School, London.

Approval for publication as a BMA policy report was recommended by the BMA Council on 6 May 1998.

2 The nature and prevalence of domestic violence

What is meant by domestic violence?

The term 'domestic violence' is used in this report to refer to physical, sexual or emotional violence from an adult perpetrator directed towards an adult victim in the context of a close relationship. Most often this will mean domestic violence from a man to his wife, ex-wife, female partner or ex-partner. This term has been adopted because it is most frequently used and is recognised in legislation, in government publications[1,2] and in common parlance. Domestic violence can include criminal and non-criminal behaviour, physical violence, psychological abuse and sexual abuse and assault (some acts of sexual abuse may fall short of being violent or criminal acts and should therefore be distinguished from sexual assault). There is no set pattern for the type of abuse used by perpetrators or for the impact which this has upon victims.* Domestic violence can range in frequency and intensity. A common factor motivating perpetrators is the use of abusive behaviour to maintain control and power over the other person.[3]

Some examples of the definitions of domestic violence are summarised in table 1, although the lists are certainly not exhaustive. It must also be remembered that not all acts of domestic violence are inherently violent and some, but not all, may constitute a criminal offence.

---

* 'Victim' is the term used in law to refer to people who suffer criminal assaults. The term, however, has been criticised because it implies passivity and it does not accurately convey the experiences of women who live with and try to overcome domestic violence on a daily basis. Some favour the term 'survivor' instead, although this may similarly give the unhelpful impression that the effects of the abuse have been overcome. Wherever possible the term 'victim' will be avoided in this report because of the negative messages conveyed.

Table 1: Definitions of domestic violence

Physical violence	
● Biting	● Bruising
● Burning	● Choking/Strangling
● Hitting	● Kicking
● Knifing	● Murder
● Punching	● Scalding
● Scratching	● Slapping
● Sleep deprivation	● Starving

Sexual abuse/assault	
● Forced sex — anal/vaginal/oral	● Urinating on
● Sexual assault using objects	● Forced tying up
● Enforced prostitution	● Forced to mimic pornography/to take part in pornography

Psychological abuse	
● Criticism	● Verbal abuse
● Isolation from family and friends/work	● Humiliation and degradation
● Extreme jealousy and possessiveness	● Financial deprivation
● Destroying personal belongings	● Forced to do menial/trivial tasks
● Made to think they are going mad	● Threats

References to perpetrators as 'men' and victims as 'women' in the report are made to reflect the most common pattern of domestic violence in contemporary society. Research reviewed in the report shows that the majority of domestic violence perpetrators are adult males and most victims are female.[4,5] This does not mean, however, that the health implications of domestic violence in same sex relationships and domestic violence from women to men does not occur and this will be considered in this report.

How prevalent is domestic violence?

Violent crimes are recognised by the current government as posing a threat to public health.[6] The British Crime Survey (BCS) is the largest source of data on crime and victimisation in the UK. The survey is generally viewed as yielding more reliable estimates of prevalence because people are asked about their experiences of crimes in the past twelve months, including the crimes which were not reported. The most recent survey, published in 1996, contains findings from interviews with a nationally representative sample of 16,348 people. Domestic violence accounted for one quarter of all the violent crimes shown in the report. The BCS data shows a clear gender pattern to violent crime. Men who are victims of violence are most at risk of violence from other men 'outside' the home. Male to male acquaintance violence accounted for 50% of all the violent attacks on men. Twelve percent of reported assaults on men were domestic violence incidents and 50% of the perpetrators were also other men in the family. The BCS shows women are most at risk of domestic violence. Forty four percent of all violent attacks on women were domestic violence incidents. Ninety percent of these incidents involved a male perpetrator's assault on a female partner or ex-partner.[7] A detailed analysis of the data on domestic violence was completed for the 1992 BCS. This shows 11% (one in nine) of the women surveyed who had lived with a male partner reported some degree of physical violence occurring during their relationships.[8] Women most at risk of domestic violence tend to be younger women below the age of 40. The reported prevalence of domestic violence decreases after the age of 40.

> ❝*Domestic violence accounted for one quarter of all violent crimes shown in the 1996 British Crime Survey*❞

The BCS is based upon a survey of people in their own homes. In this context it can be difficult for interviewers to ensure that no other household member — possibly the perpetrator of violence — is present during the interview. It also focuses only upon physical violence in the past 12 months, (being hit with fist, kicked, attacked with a weapon etc) rather than on the broader experience of violence, abuse and sexual violence over the lifespan. As a result there is a tendency for the BCS to underestimate the prevalence of the experience of domestic violence in the UK population.

Surveys which include sexual violence and a broader range of abusive behaviour show domestic violence affecting more than one in four women at some time in their lives. In 1993 a survey of 12,300 women in Canada found almost one in three (29%) had experienced violence from a current or past marital partner since the age of 16.[9] In the UK, several smaller scale local studies show similar rates of prevalence. Jayne Mooney's study in Islington, based upon interviews with 571 women and 429 men, found one in three women reported suffering domestic violence during their lives. Just under a quarter, 23%, said they had been raped (defined as 'made to have sex without consent') by their partners or ex-partners. Twelve percent (about one in nine) said they had experienced physical violence from a current or former male partner in the last 12 months.[10]

A recent study in Hackney of 129 women at GPs' surgeries and of case records held by the police, housing and social services measured the prevalence of three levels of abuse: abuse which was primarily non-physical, verbal, financial or psychological (Type A), physical abuse, such as slaps and punches (Type B), and physical and sexual abuse which was likely to require medical attention such as kicks in the face, attempted strangulation etc (Type C). This study similarly estimated the prevalence of Type C domestic violence (reported physical violence which was serious enough to need medical attention) as being one in nine during the past 12 months and almost one in three (29%) over the lifespan.[11]

Dominy and Radford's study of 484 women in Surrey found one in four of the women reported domestic violence from current and former partners during their adult lives and reported being 'forced to have sex'.[12]

Painter's study of over 1000 women gathered from 12 town centres found one in four reported an experience of marital rape.[13] In the USA, in a representative survey of 930 women in San Francisco, Dianna Russell found 12% of the 640 married women said they had been raped by their husbands.[14]

> **❝It is estimated that one in four women will experience domestic violence at some time in their lives❞**

The research findings give varied estimates of prevalence because of their varied methods of data collection and the different definitions of 'domestic violence' used. The research suggests, however, that domestic violence is both a relatively common and serious problem. Domestic violence is more likely to result in injury than any other violent crime. Sixty nine percent of domestic violence incidents result in an injury. Thirteen percent result in broken bones compared with 4% of muggings.[15] These injuries result despite the fact that weapons are used infrequently. Effective intervention and support early on is crucial because the severity of the violence has been found to escalate over time.[16]

Women are often at greater risk of violence on separation.[17] The Statistics Canada survey found that one fifth of women who experienced violence from a former partner said that the violence continued after separation. Thirty five percent of the women reported *increased* violence at that time.[18] One out of every three women living in refuges (shelters) in 1980 reported continued abuse from their ex-partners after separation.[19] Similar figures for continued domestic violence from former partners were reported by women in the BCS (36%)[20] and in Jayne Mooney's study (34%).[21] A father's continued contact with children after separation or divorce may provide a particular flash point for further violence. A qualitative study of 53 mothers recently separated from violent men found that arrangements made for children's contact with fathers after separation lead to further violence from the father for all but three of the mothers.[22] Women with children, especially women aged between 16 to 29 years are at greater risk of domestic violence.[23]

> **❝***Women with children, especially women aged between 16-29 years are at greater risk of domestic violence***❞**

A common response to domestic violence is the suggestion that the woman should leave her abuser. It is important to bear in mind that, as evidence suggests, leaving the abuser may not always bring an end to the violence.

Problems in measuring prevalence

Domestic violence is often described as a 'hidden crime'. Within the health care context it has been given little attention. Many incidents of domestic violence are unreported, not recorded or not prosecuted. Of all violent crimes, domestic violence is the least likely to come to the attention of the police or the criminal justice system.[24] The crimes which come before the courts represent the tip of the iceberg of prevalence.[25] Although studies of help seeking strategies show that the police and general practitioners are the two agencies most often approached,[26,27] information on prevalence from the police and GPs is poor.[28,29]

It is not possible to give an accurate figure for prevalence because there has never been a national study which has been able to address the problem of the under-reporting of physical and sexual abuse. Significant numbers of women do not tell anyone of their experiences of domestic violence. A study of 484 women at shopping centres in the county of Surrey found that two out of three women who had experienced domestic violence had told no one about the abuse.[30] Jayne Mooney's study of domestic violence in the North London borough of Islington found that 45% of the women who had experienced domestic violence in the past 12 months had told no one about it.[31] Women are most likely to confide in and seek support from informal networks and from their family and friends.[32,33]

An inter-agency circular on domestic violence issued by the Home Office in 1995[34] highlighted a number of reasons why an individual experiencing domestic violence might find this difficult to report to the police or other agencies. The possible reasons outlined include:

- the emotional relationship between the victim and the perpetrator;

- the perpetrator's behaviour may fluctuate between extremes;

- fear of reprisals;

- a tendency to minimise rather than exaggerate the violence and hide it from family and friends;

- pressure from the family/local community to remain in the relationship;

- worry about the effect on their children whether they stay or leave;

- financial dependence upon their partner;

- not knowing a safe place to go or the sources of help and advice available;

- a less than helpful response from agencies to whom they may have turned for help;

- repeated abuse may undermine a woman's confidence in her ability to take decisions and act.

All would similarly present barriers to the identification of domestic violence in a health care setting. The definition and recognition of an experience of violence or abuse as a 'crime' will also be an important factor influencing prevalence rates in surveys and agency statistics. The broader the definition, the higher the prevalence rates detected.[35] Police records, criminal statistics and government crime surveys all tend to undercount domestic violence because they use a narrower definition of domestic violence which is based upon acts of criminal, physical violence occurring within a limited period of time, usually within the past 12 months. Surveys of victimisation generally include a broader range of abusive behaviour; they give higher estimates of prevalence and are more likely to look at the experiences of violence over the lifespan. Findings may, however, by biased towards the views of people with an interest in the subject, particularly if the sample has been self selected.

Difficulties in undertaking research on domestic violence in health care settings

A recent editorial in the Journal of the American Medical Association[36] highlights some of the considerable difficulties encountered in trying to undertake domestic violence research. Firstly, there is no consistent definition of 'domestic' or 'violence' which means study findings are difficult to compare directly and are often not generalisable. This situation arises from different perceptions of the nature of domestic violence. Focusing on (and measuring) only abuse resulting in injury overlooks the reality of violent domestic relationships which are characterised by power and control being exerted by a man over a woman partner. Psychological abuse, threats, manipulation and coercion are for some women the most difficult aspects to contend with. Studies indicate that both physical and psychological abuse operate in most abusive relationships. Varying definitions of domestic violence contribute to the lack of a 'gold standard' for its measurement and few of the tools in use for detection are adequately validated. Nevertheless, violence inflicted towards a woman by a male partner or ex-partner is the focus of most health-based studies. This differs from some crime surveys (eg the BCS) where 'domestic violence' includes violence between any household members.

Secondly, compounding these problems, well designed, methodologically rigorous studies are the exception and sample sizes are often small. As a consequence research evidence is patchy and incomplete.[37] This also applies to studies on effective domestic violence interventions. The research that does exist is often not of high quality and unlikely to be evidence-based in the way that most medical research is conducted currently. This lack of evidence does not mean that domestic violence should be dismissed as a health care issue, but that more research is required.

3 Understanding domestic violence

The perpetrator

Knowledge about perpetrators has developed from two sources: what women say about their ex-partners' behaviour; and exceptional samples of violent men who have been sanctioned for their crimes or who are attending treatment or anti-violence programs. Most of the research on perpetrators has been completed in the USA, although there are some publications in the UK based upon the experience and observations of people working with men's groups.[1,2] Various research reports by psychologists have identified 'common characteristics' in domestic violence perpetrators, these include holding traditional views about men's position in the family, pathological jealousy, hostility to women but dependence upon the partner, low self esteem etc.[3] However, no studies have been found which attempt to compare the behaviour, attitudes and psychological profiles of abusive and non-abusive men. It is not possible to draw upon research findings to identify character traits of behaviour which could predict the likelihood of someone being an abuser. Predicting criminal behaviour from fixed personality characteristics has been notoriously time consuming and unproductive for criminologists. The emphasis in criminological thinking has now shifted onto understanding the social contexts of crime. In research on domestic violence the emphasis has shifted onto looking at the power relationships and gender issues which affect the crime. Exploring the impact which perceptions of masculinity and femininity have had upon the use of force and violence in intimate relationships has been influential in the more recent development of re-educating, behaviour challenging work with domestic violence perpetrators.

The Domestic Abuse Intervention Project in Duluth, Minnesota, USA manages one of the longest running projects working to change the behaviour of perpetrators of violence. This multi-agency intervention project has developed training materials for use in re-educative group work. The 'Power and Control' and 'Equality' wheels were devised by battered women in Duluth to help perpetrators to recognise the difference between controlling and violent behaviour and on the other hand, behaviour which is generally regarded as being more egalitarian. They are used as part of the 'Power and Control: Tactics of Men who Batter' educational curriculum. The 'Power and Control' wheel, illustrated below, identifies violent behaviour as including physical and sexual violence, coercion and threats, intimidation, emotional abuse, isolation, economic abuse, using children, using male privilege and minimizing or denying the abuse or shifting blame on to the partner.

Figure 1: Duluth model of violent behaviour[4]

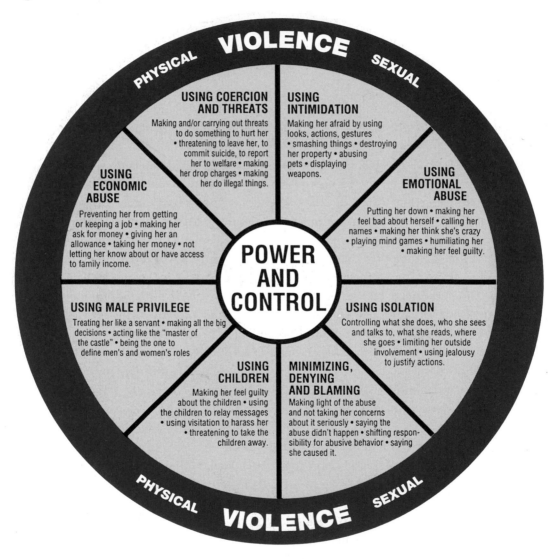

The 'Equality' wheel, illustrated below, contrasts this abusive behaviour with non-violence and non-threatening behaviour, showing respect and trust, giving support, being honest and accountable, fairly negotiating, taking shared responsibility, having economic partnership and responsible parenting.

Figure 2: Duluth model of non-violent behaviour[5]

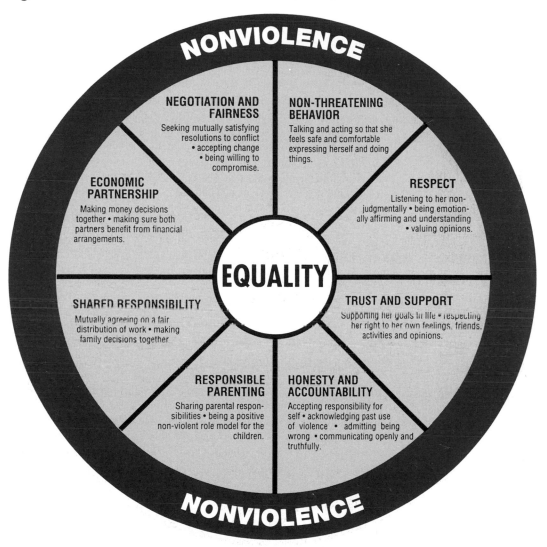

Many professionals have found the Duluth wheels helpful for pointing out the wide range of abusive and controlling behaviour used by perpetrators of domestic violence in the context of an intimate relationship where inequalities of power exist. Few perpetrators of domestic violence admit their responsibility for the violence and some are surprised to find that they may have committed a criminal offence.[6] Perpetrators often try instead to justify or excuse the violence or blame the woman for having precipitated events. Getting them to accept their own responsibility is the first objective of most re-educative anti-violence groups.[7]

For public agencies and the professions, it is important to beware of some perpetrators' propensity to involve others in their harassment campaigns. Battery by law — manipulating or abusing legal procedures and legal loopholes in order to financially and emotionally drain a former partner — has been identified as a particular problem for the courts.[8,9] The diagnostic rather than adversarial focus of the health care context gives perpetrators of domestic violence less scope for this, although they may still attempt to gain control of the medical setting by:

- **Talking for a partner and answering all the questions directed at her**, thereby ensuring that his version of events and explanation for the injuries is the only one presented. Scope to do this is enhanced if the woman lacks language skills, has a disability or depression which affects her ability to communicate.

- **Refusing to allow the woman to be seen on her own**, accompanying her into the examination room etc, so that she is unable to disclose her experiences of domestic violence.

- **Communicating directly with medical staff about his partner's health care in her absence** and giving inaccurate information, particularly about her mental health or her capacity to care for the children.

These possibilities point to the need for skilled interviewing by all health care professionals and the use of patient advocacy services for women who lack language skills.

Why do some women stay with or return to the perpetrator?

Some people can find it difficult to understand why some women stay with or return to live with abusive partners. Professionals who invest a lot of time and energy in helping women to separate from their partners can find it difficult to maintain their sympathy and understanding. Decisions which seem 'irrational' to an observer may be an understandable response for a woman who is trying to survive on a daily basis in an abusive relationship.[10] In a recent qualitative study of 22 women's experiences of surviving abusive relationships,

Glass highlights the many reasons why women do not, or feel they cannot, leave.[11] Reasons illustrated in the women's testimonies include:

- **The perpetrator not letting her go,** pursuing and harassing her, kidnapping her and forcing her to return with threat and fear. The perpetrators' pursuit of his partner may be aided and abetted by his family or friends.

- **Fear for her life**, based upon past experience and credible threats from the perpetrator. The most lethal cases of domestic violence show a pattern of escalating violence, numerous attempts by the woman to leave and a narrowing of her options to find safety.[12]

- **Feeling that it is 'all her fault'** and consequently that she has the responsibility to work at the relationship or to help the abusive partner to find a 'cure' for his violence.

- **Feelings that there is no way out**, as a result of previous attempts to leave and the lack of legal advice and law enforcement.

- **Isolation from family and friends**, usually as a result of the domestic violence combined with feelings that she cannot cope, economically or emotionally, as a single person or a single parent family.

- **Concern for the welfare of children**, fears about 'losing' children to the abusive partner, fears that social services or the courts will judge her to be an 'unfit mother', pressure from the children to return home.

- **Denial of the impact which the violence is having upon her own or her children's welfare**, there is a tendency for this denial to grow as women 'blank off' or minimalise the abuse.

- **Stigma and an unsympathetic response** from family, friends or service providers. This can be a particular problem if the violent partner has a high social status in the local community or if he is seen to be a worthy person.

- **The impact of the violence upon the woman's health**, the health aspects of domestic violence are discussed later in this report. Where the violence is adversely affecting the woman's health, service providers may see her as presenting the major problem. The effects of violence on the woman — depression, drug dependency, physical disability, chronic pain etc — can be misinterpreted as being the cause.

- **Being in love with the perpetrator** and hoping he will change.

- **The perpetrator's threats or attempts to commit suicide.**[13]

17

'Battered Women Syndrome' (BWS) was a term coined by Walker in the early 1970's[14] and is characterised by psychological, emotional and behavioural deficits arising from chronic and persistent violence. It is a syndrome that has in recent years been recognised in the British courts, is well known among agencies working with victims of domestic violence and can be a useful frame of reference in terms of understanding the victim's reactions.

The central features of BWS include 'learned helplessness', passivity and paralysis, as well as the concept of a 'Cycle of Violence' which has three phases; the 'build-up' phase, the 'impact phase' and the phase of 'contrition' and remorse, following which, the cycle starts again. Many women find it difficult to leave their partners because of their evident distress, remorse and promises to reform after having been violent and this pattern can be helpful in explaining why many women find it difficult to break away. The term 'traumatic pathological attachment' is an extreme form of co-dependency between the victim and the perpetrator, forged through fear rather than through bonds of affection, and is similar to the attachments that often develop between the hostage and kidnapper or the terrorist and the victim. It is not that the woman wishes to remain within a dangerous situation, but more likely that the alternative may be even more dangerous and uncertain. This is a useful concept in helping the health professional to understand what may appear to be a paradoxical response by the woman to her violent partner.

> **❝*It may not be that the woman wishes to remain within a dangerous situation but more likely that the alternative may be even more dangerous and uncertain*❞**

Concerns about women who return to live with violent men need to be put into proportion and considered with the considerable evidence which shows that the majority do leave and separate permanently.[15,16,17] Some may make many attempts to get out of the situation before succeeding. The main impetus to leave may not be a particular episode of violence but the realisation that things are not going to change and a growing concern that the violence, could be affecting the children.[18] Research which looks at the experiences of women who move into refuges shows women most often separate: very soon after the violence has begun; when the violence is seen to be affecting the children; and when the children are older and less dependent.[19]

Given the difficulty in separating from a violent partner and the limited options many women have available to them as single parent families, domestic violence researchers have suggested that it is more helpful to replace the question 'Why don't battered women leave?' with 'Who stops them from leaving and why do they stop them from leaving?' This would shift the emphasis on to looking in a more informed way at the effects of abuse on women and on to the social support which is available.

Is there an association between domestic violence and poverty?

Domestic violence has been found in all classes and social groups, but the available research suggests that women with lower incomes are more likely to be 'counted' as they take up residence in refuges and are more likely to turn to the public sector for help and advice.[20] In Jayne Mooney's study of domestic violence in Islington, professional women were found to be less likely to report violence to their GPs, to the police, a solicitor or any other 'outside' agency and more likely to report the abuse to friends or relatives. Twenty five percent of the professional women said they had suffered domestic violence at some time in their lives (7% in the last 12 months), whilst 30% of working class women reported an experience of violence (10% in the last 12 months). Jayne Mooney also surveyed 429 men about the use of 'conflict' in their relationships. There was little difference in the rates of *reporting* violent behaviour between professional and working class men. Twenty percent of the professional men surveyed admitted they had hit their partners compared with 21% of working class men and 17% of lower middle class men.[21]

There may be an association between domestic violence and poverty, but this does not mean there is a causal relationship between the two. The higher rates of domestic violence reported by women in lower socio-economic groups may point to, but do not necessarily lead to the conclusion that poverty breeds violence.[22,23] They do, however, indicate the difficulties many women experiencing domestic violence face in finding protection from abuse if they have low incomes.

Poverty is commonly measured at the level of the household unit. The aggregate household resources are assumed to be shared fairly between men, women and children, but this is often not the case, particularly if there is domestic violence.[24] The poverty which many women and children experience in the family because of the assumption that family finances will be fairly shared was noted over 70 years ago by the Family Allowances campaigner Eleanor Rathbone.[25] The poverty which women and children continue to suffer towards the end of this century is highlighted by the many women who report an *increase* in their standard of living when drawing Income Support after separating from a violent partner.[26] It should not be presumed that women with affluent partners or women living in affluent areas (so-called 'Middle England') necessarily have access to resources which will enable them to help themselves. Women living with affluent partners can often experience poverty because of their lack of access to the 'family' finances.

Minority groups and domestic violence

Fair access to services will be one of the six areas assessed in the proposed new system of NHS monitoring.[27] Anti-discriminatory methods of working with people affected by domestic violence and who have disabilities, from ethnic minority groups or from the gay and lesbian community are very underdeveloped in some parts of the UK.[28] It can be difficult for practitioners and service providers to obtain guidance which will help them to offer high quality services to all their clients, regardless of race, disability, age or sexual orientation. An important first step for practitioners developing equal opportunities practice is gaining knowledge about the relevant issues. The BMA has produced two reports which have made recommendations on the need for training at undergraduate and postgraduate level on disability matters[29] and on sexual orientation.[30] The following three sections briefly outline the specific issues which race and ethnicity, disability and sexual orientation raise for people who experience domestic violence.

Ethnicity, race and culture

Women from minority ethnic groups, especially those for whom English is not their first language, may find it much more difficult to get protection from domestic violence because of the poor accessibility of refuges, legal and welfare services.[31,32] Stereotypical beliefs about 'passive' Asian women or about endemic domestic violence in some communities may underlie the responses of some service providers. Feelings that the police may not give a helpful response and fears of deportation resulting from insecure immigration status have a significant impact upon the levels of reporting domestic violence amongst black women.[33]

Notions of family honour (*izzat*) and shame (*sharam*) play an important part in Asian families and can severely constrain an abused woman's ability to contact the police or social services or to separate from a violent partner. Women who have strong religious identities may find it difficult to cope without the support of their family and local community, especially if they have children.[34] Families may be unable to give support to Asian women who suffer violence because they may be seen by the rest of the community as 'interfering'. The problems some women face in separating from the abuser are compounded if his family are abusive as well. The poor accessibility of services for Asian women is further frustrated by the gatekeeping practises of some members of the police and social services, who are reluctant to intervene because they feel such matters are best dealt with 'by the community'.[35] Women from ethnic minority groups are consequently more likely to suffer domestic violence for longer because there are fewer alternatives available to them.

Health care services may be the first and only point of contact for some women from ethnic minority groups who experience domestic violence. Raising the issue and then getting access to culturally relevant services may be difficult for women whose first language is not English. Fairer access to services and fair treatment will only be possible if doctors and nurses have access to translators (other than the immediate family member) and patient advocates who have knowledge about domestic violence. The emphasis on partnership in the NHS, with local authorities and local communities, set out in the recent Green Paper, *Our Healthier Nation,*[36] may well provide a positive context for the development of these essential services and the development of best practice guidelines for doctors and inter-agency training on anti-discriminatory working.

Gay and lesbian relationships and domestic violence

Little is known about the prevalence of domestic violence in lesbian and gay relationships as crime surveys have tended to ignore this issue, and most academic research studies have been based upon small or self-selected samples of gay or lesbian abuse victims. Partner abuse does sometimes happen in gay and lesbian relationships, but it is important to be aware that this does not simply mirror the abuse found in heterosexual relationships. There are some similarities in the range and type of abusive behaviour experienced,[37] but there are also important differences in the consequences and impact in the context of a gay or lesbian relationship. The availability of services and the difficulties gay and lesbian people face as a result of discrimination presents specific problems. Disclosing an experience of violence from a partner frequently means the victim will also have to disclose his or her sexuality and thus face the risk of a homophobic reaction from the service provider. Perpetrators may also use 'homophobic control' over their partners[38] by threatening to disclose her sexuality to her family or her employer. Renzetti's research found 21% of interviewees had partners threaten to 'out' them. Fear of being 'outed' will be especially acute for gay and lesbian people who work with, or who care for children because of the false correlation often made between child abuse and sexual orientation.[39] For men in same sex relationships, fear of AIDS or suffering from AIDS can limit the man's capacity to leave an abusive partner.[40]

Domestic violence and disability

People with disabilities are at greater risk of all forms of abuse and violence than are the general population. People with disabilities are particularly vulnerable to abuse from care givers, whether in an institutional or non-institutional setting.[41] Domestic violence to people with disabilities may be more difficult to identify because the perpetrator may also be the primary care giver and will often exercise some degree of control over communication with health care workers, as well as having control over the disabled person's finances, mobility and transport opportunities. The disability may be the result of the perpetrator's abuse and if they are seen to be the primary care giver, the disabled person's dependence, isolation and entrapment in the relationship will increase. Similarly, if the perpetrator has some degree of disability and the partner is the care giver, feelings of responsibility for their care can also make it more difficult to end the abusive relationship.

Domestic violence against people with disabilities can be related to the disability itself. The abusive care giver may deny the disabled person access to the toilet, refuse help with bathing, neglect food care, take away essential walking or sensory aids or control the use of medication.[42] Poor levels of sex education, stereotypical and widely held contradictory beliefs that people with disabilities are either naively over-sexed or not aware nor concerned about sexual matters, makes women with learning difficulties particularly vulnerable to sexual abuse.[43] There is scope for much preventive work to be done in the context of sex education for disabled people and their carers.

It can be difficult for a person with disabilities to find advice or help to end the domestic violence. Katie Cosgrove and Jan Macleod interviewed women with disabilities and representatives from disability groups in Strathclyde and found numerous reports of care workers and medical staff ignoring what women said because they had decided they 'knew what was best for her'.[44] Services available to help women who experience domestic violence are seldom accessible to people with disabilities apart from within refuges and little effort has been made to make them so. Disability groups have also shown little interest in domestic violence and in the accessibility of services for people with disabilities who suffer domestic violence. People with disabilities may, as a result, be particularly dependent upon GPs and other members of the primary health care team in finding help to overcome domestic violence. Adequate training for this role and the use of advocacy services where they exist can only be beneficial for health care providers.

Commonly held unhelpful beliefs

Alcohol, drug dependency and domestic violence

A higher prevalence of alcohol consumption has often been found among perpetrators of violent crimes, particularly among younger men. 'Drinking' or drug abuse problems are often used by domestic violence perpetrators to explain or to excuse the abuse, but there is a lack of evidence to support the conclusion that these are the sole or primary causal factors.[45]

It is not possible to establish a causal relationship between alcohol abuse and domestic violence, even though some perpetrators and some victims may well have been drinking prior to an assault. Research into women's experiences of domestic violence shows that many assaults occur when the perpetrator is sober and has not taken drugs or alcohol, indeed the majority are not alcoholics nor drug abusers.[46] The British Crime Survey (BCS) found that, apart from muggings, it was less likely for domestic violence offenders to be under the influence of alcohol or drugs than for other 'contact crimes'.[47]

Women who experience domestic violence may develop alcohol dependency in response to abuse over a period of time. The American social scientists Evan Stark and Anne Flitcraft monitored the full medical histories of 481 women who sought aid for injuries from a hospital emergency room. They compared the psychosocial profiles of battered and non-battered women and they found that, apart from a small number of women who showed some alcohol dependency before the onset of domestic violence, battered women were no more likely than non-battered women to present with psychosocial problems such as drug abuse, suicide attempts or psychiatric disorders. After the first and subsequent injuries however, women showed a higher rate of diagnosis for all these psychosocial problems, including alcohol dependency. The findings were confirmed by a later study of 3,676 women visiting emergency rooms in the Yale area.[48]

In cases where a perpetrator or a victim is in need of treatment for drug or alcohol dependency problems, the pressing need to protect the victim from violence can become obscured for a variety of reasons. The symptoms may be treated (although not always) whilst their cause, the violence, stays unchecked.[49]

Violence begets violence?

It may seem reasonable to conclude that children learn about relationships on the basis of their own experiences and observations of family life, however research which has attempted to explore whether children from violent families grow up to abuse or be abused themselves is inconclusive.[50] There has been extensive research on this matter in the USA.

Many of the studies are methodologically flawed. They are based solely on unrepresentative clinical samples, they lack control groups or rely upon retrospective accounts. The definitions of 'abuse' employed vary from the very broad to more specific definitions which include children witnessing domestic violence or being physically assaulted themselves.[51] Experiencing violence in childhood may increase the risk of becoming a violent adult, but it can also lead to an abhorrence to violence and a determination not to be abusive in adult life. Indeed, most perpetrators and victims of domestic violence have been found to come from non-violent families themselves[52] and violent men share many of the character traits which are found among the non-violent population.[53] There are no specific or attitudinal characteristics which make some women more vulnerable than others to domestic violence.[54] Focusing too much upon the difficulties adults may have suffered as children can detract from the more immediate need for intervention to stop current violent behaviour.

Gender, equality and violence

Notions of femininity do not deter women from committing homicides nor gross acts of cruelty and abuse. The extent to which women use violence in the family or towards partners has been a subject of particular interest to the media in recent times. Much of the debate has been based upon speculation about women's liberation and the breaking down of 'traditional thinking' about what men and women can do. It has been argued that domestic violence to men happens just as frequently as domestic violence to women, but this is not openly talked about nor brought to the attention of the courts because of men's greater feelings of shame and stigma.[55,56] There is little doubt that men, like women who suffer abuse, experience feelings of shame and may be reluctant to talk about the experience and be fearful of seeking help. Finding ways to break down the barriers so that people who suffer violence feel safe to seek help from health care providers and relevant agencies is an important issue which will be considered further in this report. However, acknowledging that men and women can bully and dominate their partners does not mean that the gendered aspect of domestic violence should be ignored because this has a very major impact upon the social context of the crime. Ignoring this social context would mean taking a step backwards from current policies which have started to tackle some of the social, economic, cultural and institutional factors which affect violent crime. The evidence available from the range of domestic violence research studies conducted over the past 25 years does not support the idea that there is a 'gender equality' in the use or experience of violence. The findings do support the conclusion that violence committed by both men and women is strongly influenced by our thinking about gender.

The claim that there is an 'equality in violence' is generally based on three main sources of data: the first National Survey on Family Violence in the USA; a MORI poll commissioned for the BBC documentary programme *Here and Now* and the findings from the British Crime Survey (BCS). The findings from the BCS have already been mentioned in this report, 145,000 or so of these incidents of domestic violence to men were reported as being violence from women to men (about 6% of all the assaults on men). A more detailed analysis of the domestic violence findings from the 1996 BCS will soon be available.[57] It would be useful to have an analysis which sheds light on the debates about the degree to which men and women differ in the use of violence. At present there is no way of determining from the BCS figures the proportion of assaults by men upon men which took place in the context of an intervention by a son, new partner or other family member to protect or deter an attack upon a woman. Nor is it possible to assess the degree to which women use violence against men to defend themselves or other family members and the degree to which violence is used as a direct attack. Homicide research shows a gendered pattern in the use of lethal violence. Men are less often victims of women's lethal violence and more likely to be killed by other men they know. Each year, 45% of female homicide victims in England and Wales are killed by present or former male partners, compared to 8% of male victims killed by current or former female partners.[58] The motivation for homicides of adults has been shown to vary for men and women. The majority of domestic homicides by men are preceded by disputes over sexual jealousy. Men most frequently kill their partners because they fear or suspect the woman's infidelity. A highly important risk factor in homicide for women is separation or divorce.[59] Women who kill partners do so mostly in the context of a self defence against a man's battery.[60]

The extent to which women initiate violence has been a topic of some controversy in the USA research on family violence. The first National Survey on Family Violence in the USA in 1975 was based upon a representative questionnaire survey of 2,143 husbands and wives. The survey found that 11.6% of wives admitted using 'violence' against their husbands and 12.1% of husbands admitted using 'violence' to wives.[61] The more recent *Here and Now* MORI poll in England concluded that women were more likely than men to be violent to their partners. The MORI poll and the National Family Violence survey measured 'conflict', not only violence, using a research instrument called the Conflict Tactics Scale (CTS). The early application of the scale brought heavy criticisms from the academic community and it has since been developed and refined. A very crude version of this scale was employed in the MORI poll survey and it has been similarly criticised.[62] The CTS, as used in these surveys, applied a one dimensional measure of conflict resolution tactics to ask spouses how they dealt with family disputes. The full scale measures tactics ranging from life threatening violence — using a knife or weapon — to avoidance tactics such as walking out of the room. Sexual violence was not included in the scale, so a potentially large range of abusive behaviour which men more commonly employ was excluded from both surveys. The scale measures the frequency of events, but the 1975 survey and MORI poll research did not put these into context nor look at the consequences of the use of violence by men and women. It is not possible to tell from the results yielded whether or not 'violent' acts reported took place in the context of an attack or a defence. Nor is it possible to explore the consequences and harm which resulted. The ranking of violence within the scale has been argued to be meaningless without some reference to context and consequence.[63] A 'slap' from a large and muscular man which resulted in a woman losing her teeth could be ranked as less violent than a battered woman picking up a knife in a desperate and futile attempt to prevent another assault. Categories such as 'threw something at spouse' might include throwing a cushion and throwing a chair. The MORI poll placed particular emphasis upon 'verbal violence' which similarly could include a huge range of violent, abusive and irritating behaviour as well as inviting biased responses about partners who 'nag'.

The second national family violence survey in 1985 attempted to address these criticisms by following up the use of the CTS with supplementary questions about the context of the abuse. 6002 individuals were surveyed and more than one in four of them (28%) reported experiencing domestic violence in their marriages. Taking the context and consequences of abuse into account, the leading American family violence researchers drew very different conclusions about gender and violence. Domestic violence from women to men (ie where women were the primary aggressors and violence was the result) was said to have occurred in 4% of the families surveyed. The most common pattern for domestic violence was found to be violence from men to women.[64]

The controversy over the American family violence research highlights the potential difficulties in identifying and acting upon reports of domestic violence if the social context of the crime is ignored. Faced with allegations and counter-allegations, doctors and GPs are in favourable positions for gaining information on the context of violent events. Doctors and GPs have access to information on the harm caused to victims in the form of medical evidence. The privacy of the medical setting usually means that they will be in a position to directly ask patients about abuse. Twenty five years of research into domestic violence has brought guidance for doctors and GPs on how to ask patients about abuse (this will be discussed in Chapter Six).

It is regrettable that the data that exists on violence to men has not been used more constructively to inform work with victims of violence. Most often the gender equality arguments have been used either to deny the need to provide services to protect women and children from domestic violence, or to raise arguments about false allegations of violence in court proceedings affecting children.[65] It is quite likely that men who suffer domestic violence find it hard to get their fears taken seriously, but claims made that there is a huge potential demand for services from battered men are not convincing in light of the fact that services set up to cater for men's needs have closed down due to lack of demand.[66] Refuge services for women and children are, on the other hand, constantly over-stretched by the demand.[67]

4 The impact of domestic violence upon health

The impact which domestic violence has will vary from person to person, but it has a major impact on health which extends well beyond physical injury alone.[1] There is growing evidence to confirm that domestic violence does have serious and long lasting consequences for the well-being of women and children. There has been no research to date which comprehensively addresses both the short and long term (lifetime) costs which domestic violence has for women and children, although there are now recent studies in the UK which have considered the health consequences, the costs to services and the impact upon the welfare of children.[2,3]

The two most important health consequences of domestic violence are the physical injury (including sexual abuse) and the psychological effects.

Physical injury

Physical violence is typically ongoing and repeated and the range of injury is wide. Unlike women injured by other means, those assaulted by a partner or ex-partner are thirteen times more likely to be injured in the breast, chest and abdomen.[4] Pregnancy is a time when abuse may start or escalate. A wide range of prevalence of domestic violence during pregnancy is reported from 0.9% to over 20% depending on the study methodology[5] and injury to the abdomen, breasts and genital area is common at this time.[6] Women may be at even higher risk in the postpartum period[7] and miscarriage and low birth weight babies are more common in abused women.[8,9] A survey of 127 women living in refuges in Northern Ireland found that 60% reported violence and abuse during pregnancy, 13% lost babies as a result and 22% reported a threatened loss of their babies.[10] Injuries which can result from violence during pregnancy include placental separation, foetal fractures, rupture of the uterus and pre-term labour. Poor diet and restricted access to ante-natal care also has some impact, as yet not fully explored, upon the health of mothers and children.[11]

A recent study of 1750 police records of domestic violence incidents in the Hackney area found one in four of the incidents reported resulted in substantial physical injuries (attempts to kill, strangulation, stabbing, broken bones or attempts to set fire to the other person). The same study's survey of 129 women at a GPs surgery found that 10% of the women had been knocked unconscious, 5% sustained broken nose, jaw or cheekbone and 2% broken arms, legs or ribs. On average, each woman reported having suffered more than four of these substantial injuries.[12]

A qualitative study of 56 women's experiences of domestic violence in Northern Ireland found 39% of the women interviewed (recruited through women's refuges) had, at least once, suffered violence which required hospital treatment.[13] Eleven percent (53) of the 484 surveyed in the Surrey research reported having been beaten up and 5% (20) had been attacked with a weapon.[14]

Sexual abuse

Violence against the woman is frequently directed at the genitalia and can be accompanied by sexual acts and assault which can include rape, buggery and inserting objects into the vagina or anus. In a study of 168 victims attending a medical rape trauma service in 1987 in Oslo, Norway, 4% had been raped by their partner and all had serious injuries.[15] Eighty percent of these battered women endured many violent episodes before seeking medical treatment.

It is thought that the vast majority of sexual assault cases are not reported to the police and domestic or spousal rape is even less commonly reported.[16] Until 1991, married women had no legal redress against a husband's rape, but in 1991, the House of Lords ruled that the three hundred year old rule was no longer good law.

Health care professionals should be aware and recognise that rape victims may experience 'Rape Trauma Syndrome' after the assault. This involves two defined phases; a short term phase of disbelief and shock and longer term reactions of anxiety and depression.[17] Sexual abuse can therefore have a significant impact upon the health and welfare of a women experiencing domestic violence.

Psychological effects

As well as physical injury, domestic violence can also have psychological effects including depression, anxiety, post traumatic stress disorder and suicide. Women may also feel anxious, helpless, afraid, demoralised, ashamed and angry and may experience panic attacks.[18] Battered Women Syndrome (BWS) is a psychological condition that is characterised by psychological, emotional and behavioural deficits arising from chronic and persistent violence. The central features of BWS include 'learned helplessness', passivity and paralysis.[19] Understanding BWS can be a useful frame of reference in terms of understanding the victims' reaction to domestic violence.

Post traumatic stress disorder (PTSD) refers to a range of psychological responses in people exposed to traumatic and life threatening experiences, including military combat, natural disasters, terrorist attacks, rape and inter-personal violence. In relation to domestic violence, common features associated with PTSD include anxiety, fear, experiencing flashbacks or persistently re-experiencing the event, nightmares, sleeplessness, exaggerated startle response, difficulty in concentrating, feelings of shame, despair and hopelessness.[20] There is little doubt that psychiatric illness, particularly PTSD, depression and anxiety is greater among women who have experienced domestic violence compared to those that have not.[21]

In a study of American psychiatric in-patients, 64% of women disclosed a history of physical abuse as an adult and 38% gave a history of sexual abuse as an adult, with the two tending to occur together.[22] Compared with women who have not experienced domestic violence, the prevalence of mental health problems appears to increase around the time that the violence is occurring, as well as in the longer term when the violence has ceased.[23]

In the longer term, and after separation, women most frequently stress the impact which living through domestic violence has had upon their mental health, their self esteem, feelings of self worth and security. There is a tendency to stress the psychological effects as being the most profound, even where there has been life threatening or disabling physical violence from the perpetrator.[24,25,26]

The impact that trauma can have upon mental and emotional health is recognised in the diagnosis of psychiatric disorders such as PTSD and BWS.[27] Traumatic pathological attachment, a characteristic of BWS is an extreme form of co-dependency between the victim and the perpetrator, and is forged through bonds of fear rather than through bonds of affection. This fear can restrict and limit women's lives and can compound the isolation which may result from sustained abuse.[28] Fear can mean reliving the event or having a physical reaction, such as nausea, which is triggered by an event or experience which has become associated with the abuse. The following extracts from interviews with survivors gives an impression of the impact of fear:

> *"I'm still very anxious that I don't meet him, it's almost been two years now but I'm still sort of, if I hear a motorbike pull up outside or something, I'm almost reaching for the telephone to phone the police. If I'm in the street and I hear a motorbike, I'm still trying to dive for cover"*

"You just never knew what was going to happen and when and afterward, if somebody brushes past you in the street, it gives you a fright...if somebody reaches out to touch you, you draw back. You just don't want to be touched by anybody".[29]

Rates of drug and alcohol abuse seem to rise after the first episode of violence has presented and may be a consequence of this.[30,31] Stark and Flitcraft (1996) found that women who had been abused were:

- 15 times more likely to abuse alcohol

- 9 times more likely to abuse drugs

- 3 times more likely to be diagnosed as depressed or psychotic

- 5 times more likely to attempt suicide

They also found that one in seven battered women were institutionalised in psychiatric hospitals, or received psychiatric referrals, yet no incidence of domestic violence was recorded on their referral notes.[32]

"75-90% of most domestic violence incidents are witnessed by children"

The impact upon children

Domestic violence to the mother is very likely to have some effect upon the welfare of children. In households where there are children, most domestic violence incidents (75 to 90%) are witnessed by the children, although adults may not always be aware that the children have been present or have heard what has happened from an adjacent room.[33] Witnessing domestic violence can cause considerable harm to children in both the short and long term. In the short term, both boys and girls who have witnessed domestic violence may show a range of disturbed behaviour, including withdrawal, depression, increased aggression, fear and anxiety. Boys are more likely to show increased aggression in the longer term. The signs children exhibit vary in relation to their ages, gender and development.[34] Psychologists in Canada estimate that half of the children living in women's shelters (refuges) are likely to show signs of PTSD.[35]

Children who witness domestic violence may blame themselves for it happening, or take on responsibility to protect the mother and/or siblings.[36,37] Children may feel guilty that they were unable to protect their mothers and to stop the violence from happening. Fathers sometimes make attempts to implicate the children in the abuse of the mother and thereby compound a child's feelings of guilt or responsibility. This can have a poor effect upon the relationship between the child and the mother. After a divorce or separation, the father often has contact/access to the child without adequate supervision so that it can be particularly difficult to thwart his attempts to implicate the child in the abuse of the mother. Getting the child to relay threats, to 'spy' on the mother or to disclose her new address are common tactics violent men use to regain control over women who leave them.[38] Women frequently make decisions to separate from a violent partner because of concerns for the welfare of their children[39] so it is ironic that it may be through their children that some are forced to return.

Domestic violence can adversely affect the mother's capacity to parent effectively in the short and longer term.[40] There has not been sufficient research to draw any firm conclusions about the combined effects which health problems, deprivation and social isolation caused by abuse have upon parenting. The welfare of children may well be adversely affected by a range of other hardships associated with domestic violence — social isolation, restrictions on their activities and friendships, frequent changes of residence, disruptions to their schooling, and poverty.[41]

Where there is domestic violence to the mother there is an increased risk that there will be violence to the child as well. In the USA, an association of between 45% to 70% has been found between the father's violence to the mother and his violence to the children.[42,43] Wide variations in the findings exist because of the different definitions of 'child abuse' used and because of differences between the sample populations (the samples are drawn from two main sources, women living in shelters or child abuse cases).

❝*An association of between 45-70% has been found between the father's violence to the mother and his violence to the children*❞

In the UK, studies of child protection records indicate at least a third of the children were living with mothers who had been subject to violence and abuse from their male partners.[44,45] Research by Hester and Pearson of the National Society for the Prevention of Cruelty to Children (NSPCC) child abuse case records in one locality found that in one in every three child abuse cases (mostly child sexual abuse) there were reports of domestic violence from the perpetrator to the mother as well. This rose to nearly two thirds of cases after the NSPCC team started domestic violence monitoring, showing a correspondence between child abuse and domestic violence.[46] The NSPCC has recently launched a new campaign on the link between child abuse and domestic violence. This comes after the charity analysed its records and found that of more than 2,000 live abuse cases on its teams books, one in five also involved domestic violence. It is thought the true correlation may be even higher; although the national average was 21%, as many as 32% of abuse cases being handled by teams in Wales and the Midlands had a domestic violence component also.

The charity has produced 250,000 credit card sized 'calls cards' for women and children who may be at risk. These give details of telephone helplines (see contact list at back of report) and advice services, and will be distributed to health visitors, nurses and GPs to hand out discreetly to patients who could benefit.[47]

Smaller, qualitative studies in the UK also indicate some correspondence between violence to the child and violence to the mother. A study sponsored by the NCH Action for Children surveyed 103 mothers who had suffered domestic violence visiting their family centres. 27% of the mothers said their partners had also abused the children.[48] A study of child contact arrangements and domestic violence found 21 out of 53 women participants in England reported physical or sexual violence from the partner to the child as well.[49]

The research studies which have looked at women leaving violent relationships show that many mothers make great efforts to protect their children from the father's violence.[50] Many women fear inappropriate or insensitive action from social workers or other professionals exercising their child protection responsibilities.[51] Recent publications conclude that providing support for the mother as well as ensuring the safety of the child can be a highly effective child protection strategy where there has been domestic violence.[52,53]

Child protection figures indicate that women are also violent, abusive or neglectful towards their children, but little is known about the relationship between maternal violence and domestic violence. Professionals who are able to develop their knowledge and understanding of domestic violence and its impact upon women and children will be in a better position both to protect children and provide appropriate support to parents.

The impact which domestic violence has on children varies from child to child. Children will be affected differently because their own resources and capacities to cope will vary. Having a good relationship with one caring parent (usually the mother), a supportive relationship with other significant adults, friends or relatives may also help the child to cope with witnessing and living through domestic violence.[54]

Children and domestic violence

- Where there is domestic violence to the mother there is an increased risk that there will also be physical or sexual violence to the child.[55,56]

- In households where there are children present, most domestic violence incidents are witnessed by children.[57]

- Witnessing domestic violence can cause considerable short term and long term harm.[58]

- In the short term both boys and girls may show a range of disturbed behaviour including withdrawal, depression, increased aggression, fear and anxiety.[59]

- The signs children show vary in relation to their ages, gender and development.[60]

- Children may blame themselves for the violence or take on responsibility to 'manage' the violence or to protect their mother and siblings.[61]

- Fathers may try to involve the children in the abusive behaviour, compounding the child's feelings of guilt and sometimes affecting the relationship between child and mother.[62]

- Children are especially vulnerable to abuse or manipulation by the father during poorly supervised contact meetings after the parents have separated.[63]

- Domestic violence may affect the mother's capacity to parent.[64]

- Children's welfare, social networks, education and emotional security can be adversely affected by the poverty and residential insecurity many families living through domestic violence face.[65]

The economic costs of domestic violence

Attempts have been made in the USA and in Australia to estimate the economic costs of domestic violence to public agencies over a woman's lifetime, and the costs for employers for days lost through sick leave and absenteeism.[66] Recent research in the UK has started to count the costs which domestic violence has for public services. A study by Stanko, Crisp, Hale and Lucraft of domestic violence in the London Borough of Hackney estimated the overall cost of domestic violence to public agencies in the borough as being **over £5 million** in 1996. The costs to the health services of providing treatment for injuries and psychological harm, excluding the costs of medicines and hospitalisation, were estimated to be £590,000 in Hackney and £189 million in Greater London. The costs for social services work were estimated as being £2,360,000.[67] The economic costs for individuals have never been calculated, although the review of poverty and domestic violence later in this report suggests a substantial impact which, given the association between poverty and health, will inevitably have health implications.

Cost and consequences of domestic violence

● One in four incidents result in substantial physical injuries.[68]

● A study of 129 women at GPs surgeries in Hackney found 10% had been knocked unconscious, 5% sustained broken bones as a result of domestic violence.

● On average each woman reported having suffered more than four of these injuries.[69]

● 60% of 127 women resident in refuges in Northern Ireland experienced violence during pregnancy, 13% lost their babies as a result.[70]

● In the longer term, survivors most frequently stress the psychological effects even where there has been life threatening or disabling violence.[71]

● The overall financial costs of domestic violence to public services in one London borough were estimated as being £5 million in 1996.

● The costs of providing treatment for injuries and psychological harm were estimated as being £590,000 in Hackney in 1996 and £189m in Greater London.

● The costs for social services were estimated as being £2,360,000.[72]

5 Identifying domestic violence in health care settings

Perhaps surprisingly, given reservations previously described about methodology, most prevalence studies in the USA indicate that around a quarter of women have experienced domestic violence from a male partner or ex-partner.[1] However, domestic violence is not identified at this rate in health care settings. The evidence for this lack of identification comes both from doctors and from women themselves, but the quality of this evidence is sometimes poor. This chapter will examine why many patients who experience domestic violence go undetected in health care settings, and will advise on how identification may be improved. It will be discussed in the context of a primary health care setting, but it is essential to remember that this advice applies to all health care professionals.

Doctors' behaviour and attitudes

There are a number of reasons why doctors do not identify all women who have experienced domestic violence. Some of these relate to issues of clinical practice and may therefore be amenable to change, but some also link with general attitudes to domestic violence which are perhaps more difficult to alter. Possibly the largest study of family doctors' attitudes published so far is a national survey undertaken in Canada, 963 out of a possible 1574 eligible to respond to a mailed questionnaire did so. Around 90% of respondents believed that family doctors should diagnose 'wife abuse' in their practices. However, fewer than one third believed that family doctors are able to effectively diagnose physical abuse and even fewer believed that they could diagnose emotional abuse effectively. Almost all believed that they are missing cases of abuse and just over half of respondents estimated that they are missing 30% or more of cases. Two thirds reported not having a standard method for detecting 'wife abuse'. The reasons given most commonly for not identifying domestic violence included infrequent patient visits, unresponsiveness of patient to questions, no patient initiative, lack of time, not trained, unresponsiveness of patient to referrals and forgot to ask. Of 21 reasons for not identifying, the two least common were "it is not a medical matter" and "none of my business". Almost all felt that their most important role was in providing the woman with information concerning community resources, providing emotional support and arranging referrals. 87% believed that more educational courses on 'wife abuse' were required.[2]

Two smaller studies shed further light on factors that may contribute to lack of identification of women who have experienced domestic violence. One of these is an interview study of a selected group of primary care doctors.[3] Repeatedly the image of Pandora's box is used by the doctors to describe their fears or experiences of exploring the issues of domestic violence. Lack of time was identified by nearly three quarters of doctors as a barrier to identification. Worries were also expressed about offending the woman and jeopardising the doctor-patient relationship. Feeling powerless, not being able to fix the situation and loss of control were described. Identifying too closely with patients from a similar background may also impede identification. Another study in Canada of 32 family doctors participating in focus groups also identified lack of medical school training about 'wife abuse' and lack of knowledge about community resources as a problem for them.[4]

The medical model of care in which student doctors are traditionally educated may have a significant impact on how often domestic violence is identified, as well as the doctors' subsequent response.[5,6] This model focuses on objectivity and placing patients in a diagnostic category for which there is a defined treatment. The emphasis on objective findings such as trauma may, in the case of domestic violence, result in the true cause of the woman's symptoms being obscured. This can be a particular problem in accident and emergency settings. In a study of emergency room charts, the problem of ongoing domestic violence was mentioned in the discharge diagnosis in only 1 out of 52 cases in which abuse was explicit or strongly indicated. In three quarters of cases the doctor failed to record the relationship of the assailant to the woman.

Women's views of doctors

The way in which a woman approaches contact with her doctor may determine whether or not a history of domestic violence is identified, and so will the interaction itself. This is an area in which a substantial body of research has been produced in the UK. A study undertaken in a refuge in the late 1970's found that 32 out of 50 women had talked to their GP about domestic violence.[7] Over half had found the response helpful which was characterised by the doctor listening, being sympathetic and offering appropriate advice. General practitioners who were said to be unhelpful frequently prescribed antidepressants and tranquilisers. A later study found that 89% of women living in refuges had consulted their general practitioner in the previous year, but nearly half of these had not disclosed domestic violence, mostly because they were ashamed or were afraid their partner would find out, but also because of an unsympathetic or hurried attitude from the doctor.[8] Other studies of women in refuges found that only a quarter to a half of women had mentioned violence to their GP or contacted them for help.[9,10] A more recent community based study found that far fewer women who had experienced domestic violence or violence from another household member had approached their GP for help — only 14%. However, leaving aside friends and family, GPs were the second most likely group to be approached for help, after police, and most of the support received was described as helpful.[11] Mooney found that GPs were the statutory agency most likely to be approached for help.[12]

Another community survey found that 20% of those who sought help for violence from a known man approached the GP first (after family and friends), although only 36% of women in the sample who had experienced domestic violence sought any help at all. Eighty one percent of women found the response of GPs or health visitors helpful. Comments were made by some women that health professionals had not sufficiently probed to find the reason that help was being requested. Some GPs had only offered tranquilisers or sleeping tablets and not provided help with accessing counselling or a support group which women wanted.[13] A recent Australian study showed that the main reason women did not discuss violence with their doctor was because they were not asked.[14]

It is not known whether the gender of the health professional will have an impact on the readiness of a woman to disclose domestic violence. Research on other gender-based violence, for example rape, suggests that choice and control are the most important issues for women being seen. Beyond that it is the knowledge, understanding and sympathetic attitude shown by the doctor, rather than their gender that makes a difference.[15] Mezey *et al* also found that women attending GP's surgeries were more likely to disclose domestic violence to their health visitor, although it is unclear whether this was related to the fact that health visitors were more likely to be female, or to their different approaches to the woman.[16]

The picture that emerges overall is somewhat mixed . When women seek help from statutory agencies, the GP is likely to be high up the list of those approached. However, the number of women seeking help from their GP is not clear and the helpfulness of the GP is variable.

The health and social costs and consequences of domestic violence have already been detailed, and are extensive. Although some critics would argue against the 'medicalisation' of domestic violence, this is an issue which significantly affects the mental and physical health of large numbers of women and their children. Doctors and other health professionals are therefore inevitably involved in providing care for individuals affected by domestic violence. Identification of these women is the first step towards ensuring appropriate care.

Should all patients be asked about domestic violence?

An American study showed that the majority of women surveyed favoured routine inquiry about physical or sexual abuse (including abuse in childhood). The study included both abused and non-abused women. However, around two thirds of a small sample of doctors surveyed in the same study felt that physical and sexual abuse enquiry should not occur routinely at annual examinations.[17] Two thirds of a group of women questioned in Northern Ireland thought that doctors should ask directly about violence, and women in this group wanted to receive advice and information about what they could do and where they could go.[18] A recent study of the prevalence of any form of assault during the previous year amongst attendees at a large general practice found that 61% of men and women would disclose the incident to their GP if asked.[19] Thus, the small amount of evidence available suggests that practitioners favour a clinically triggered approach and women a routine questioning approach.

The American Medical Association guidelines on domestic violence and a large number of other North American guidelines[20] recommend that the doctor should routinely ask all women direct, specific questions about abuse. This can be justified by a recognition of the significance of domestic violence as a widespread, often hidden, health problem and evidence that an important reason why women do not discuss the issue is because they are not asked. In addition, the associated clinical features lack specificity and cannot be relied on as the only means to identify women who have experienced domestic violence. It must be recognised that such recommendations may reflect a different approach to obligatory reporting in different jurisdictions.

British guidelines implemented in health care settings are not common and tend to shy away from recommending routine questioning, instead preferring to suggest that doctors and others should maintain a high level of awareness and ask if the clinical presentation is suggestive. This includes questioning in situations where there are behavioural clues — for example when a woman's story of how an injury happens seems inconsistent, or when the woman is accompanied by an 'overprotective' partner (although asking in his presence may not be appropriate).[21]

Whether routine questioning is considered effective and appropriate would clearly depend on the questions asked and the way in which the issue of domestic violence was raised in any research. Many women, on learning of the high rate of undisclosed domestic violence, would support greater openness of this issue between doctor and patient and would agree that patients who are suffering from domestic violence should ideally expect that this matter will be raised by their doctor. This is clearly not the same, however, as supporting the proposal that at every consultation, regardless of the complaint, women patients are asked about possible domestic violence. Studies will therefore need to be carefully worded.

On the counterside it may not be necessarily helpful to rely on studies undertaken in America where patients are likely to have different characteristics and expectations from their doctors than their British counterparts. Reactions from various women patients in the UK in response to questioning about their private lives by their doctors could be very different to the attitudes of women in the United States.

While routine questioning would be likely to produce more accurate statistics on the prevalence of domestic violence, there is the possibility that questions about a patient's personal circumstances, when it is not apparently clinically indicated, might well be considered inappropriate and may on some occasions induce a greater reserve in the patient. Such enquiries could potentially damage the doctor-patient relationship if raised in an insensitive manner where the patient begins to resent the line of questioning taken by the doctor. The need for a discussion about confidentiality prior to questioning about domestic violence also raises the issue of time. There is a danger that routine questioning could become too routine with a risk that the questioning becomes purely procedural, without necessarily conveying the impression that the doctor has the time to cope with a full discussion following any disclosure. Nevertheless, studies may show in time that women patients in the UK would not object to being asked routinely about violence if it is raised in an appropriate and sensitive manner.

The evidence in support of routine questioning of all women patients is limited and further research is required in this area to determine a practice that is acceptable to both doctors and to women and is sensitive to different areas and cultures. As in many areas of medicine, in the BMA's view, and until evidence can clearly point to the most effective practice, doctors should consider what is appropriate for each patient. There should be greater focus on training and educating doctors to enable them to detect the physical and mental symptoms which may indicate domestic violence.

The need for education and training

No formal studies have been undertaken nationally in the UK on the extent of education received on domestic violence by medical students and doctors at undergraduate or post-graduate level. By contrast, a survey ten years ago of accredited USA and Canadian medical schools found that just under half of those who replied were providing some instruction on domestic violence, although the time allocated was small.[22]

By 1994, 87% of US medical schools devoted some curricular time to dealing with adult domestic violence.[23] In the UK, a recent survey of 254 GPs in the Midlands found that

10% had received some training either at undergraduate or post graduate level on domestic violence.[24]

However, the lack of formal data does not necessarily equate with an absence of teaching and learning on the issue of domestic violence in UK medical schools and in other health settings. The provision of training for health professionals on domestic violence forms an essential part of any policy which aims to improve the health of women: good examples of this exist in Glasgow and Leeds and there are others. In Greater Glasgow, implementing a women's health policy included the production of an open learning pack by one of the local hospital accident and emergency departments, to be used in conjunction with implementing a protocol on domestic violence.[25]

This seems an area which is particularly suitable for multi-professional educational initiatives which can be linked with the development of guidelines. Guidelines may increase the identification of women experiencing domestic violence[26] and can help standardise good practice, which will largely be based on local consensus. Inter-agency guidelines can help pull together professionals involved in helping women who have experienced domestic violence. However, ongoing commitment to the implementation of guidelines and to staff training is required: regular audit of process outcomes and rates of identification may be useful in this respect.

Teaching specifically directed to the needs of doctors in training is fairly well established in North America. *Academic Medicine*, the journal of the association of American medical colleges, recently produced a 115 page supplement entirely devoted to the subject of educating the nation's doctors about family violence and abuse.[27] Some of this teaching and training can be evidence-based: for example enough is known about the way abused women wish to be treated by their doctors, and the way that doctors do treat them, to inform doctors' behaviour. In the same edition of *Academic Medicine*, Warshaw highlights some of the important aspects of learning about domestic violence, including the need to acquire new knowledge and skills whilst confronting existing beliefs that shape responses to patients, and learning to work in partnership with community groups.[28]

There is also a need for teachers to model non-abusive behaviours in all aspects of training and medical care and the importance of providing a safe and supportive environment for those students who may themselves have been abused.[29] The skills required to teach this difficult and sensitive area may already exist within UK medical schools, but many Women's Aid groups and other voluntary agencies provide training on helping women who have experienced domestic violence as part of their core work.

As with much domestic violence research, measuring outcomes from training and generalising results is not easy. A detailed analysis suggests that students at UCLA developed a significant increase in their feeling of self efficacy with respect to dealing with women who have experienced domestic violence after participating in a module on domestic violence, in comparison with a group of control students.[30]

However, a study of a small number of doctors found that those who had undertaken brief training on domestic violence did not differ on any outcome variable.[31] Another study of a small number of emergency department doctor house staff showed a positive response to training on violence against women.[32]

Research already outlined indicates that doctors want to receive more training on domestic violence and that women do not always get the care that they would like from their doctors for this very common problem. These findings show education is not clear, this may be because the outcomes being measured are not appropriate or simply that the quality of education being provided needs improvement.

These findings have significant implications for both undergraduate and postgraduate medical education, in terms of highlighting its need and addressing the form and content. A greater awareness and understanding of the complexity of domestic violence and social factors which may impact on health long term is required. There is a real risk, however, of reinventing the wheel: plenty of materials, resources and experience already exist so this should be avoided.

6 Advice on good practice for identifying and dealing with domestic violence

Asking the question

How to ask questions about domestic violence is not clear but several general 'lead in' questions have been suggested, which include questions about whether the woman has ever been physically hurt by her partner or ex-partner or forced to have sex with him.[1] Others include questions about the woman's perception of her safety[2] and may include questions about whether she is afraid of her partner.

Examples of questions could include:

- Do you ever feel afraid of your partner?

- Has your partner or ex-partner ever physically hurt or threatened you?

- Has your partner ever destroyed things that you cared about?

- Has you partner ever threatened or abused your children?

- Has your partner ever forced you to have sex?

- Has your partner ever prevented you from doing things — for example leaving the house, seeing friends etc?[3]

It must be remembered that the doctor or other health professional does not necessarily need to prove the existence of domestic violence (perhaps unlike members of the legal profession), or to measure changes in the severity and frequency of the violence over time (which some therapists and others working with men may wish to do), or even to accurately detect the true prevalence of domestic violence within a particular community, but instead needs to identify and acknowledge that domestic violence is occuring.

It is essential that confidentiality is discussed in detail with the patient on each occasion that the issue of domestic violence is raised. The doctor should explain that any information provided by the patient relating to domestic violence will be treated as confidential. However, the doctor should also explain that secrecy can not always be guaranteed and that there may be rare and exceptional circumstances when the doctor may be required to breach confidentiality, for example, where children are potentially at risk or where the doctor considers that the patient, herself, may be at risk of serious harm or death (please refer to the section on confidentiality on page 51 for a detailed discussion).

A risk assessment of the woman's situation should ideally be carried out. Given that around 40% of women are murdered by an intimate partner or ex-partner, it is important to recognise situations in which the domestic violence appears to be escalating and to be able to advise the women if a lethal outcome appears likely. Factors that have been identified as predicting homicidal outcome include, rising severity and frequency of domestic violence, sexual assault (in addition to physical violence), alcohol or drugs use by the perpetrator and past suicidal attempts by the woman.[4]

If a woman feels that she is in a supportive environment, she may feel more willing to disclose domestic violence. To this end, it may be helpful to display posters and other material in the surgery about where women can get help with domestic violence. These could also be in private areas such as consulting rooms and toilets.

Women from ethnic minority groups

Women whose first language is not English, may find it difficult to access health care. Advocacy services are often inadequate and some health service advocates are men. Children or partners are not infrequently called on to interpret. It is even less likely that women in these circumstances will disclose a history of domestic violence, even though domestic violence is common in ethnic minority communities.[5] Some cultural factors may also affect women's responses to violence, and there may seem to her to be no acceptable alternatives to it.[6] Perhaps the best a GP can do is to have material available in the surgery in appropriate languages detailing relevant local resources — for example, refuges for Asian women — and to use advocates when these are available. Looking for indicators of violence may be more important if there are fewer opportunities for asking, and other members of the primary care team may have an important role to play in this respect, such as midwives or health visitors who may have regular access to the woman's home.

What to do following a disclosure

A four step action list following a disclosure of domestic violence was suggested by Heath in 1992 which included, respect and validation, assessment and medical treatment, information giving and follow up.[7,8,9]

Respect and validation

The woman's description of what has happened to her should be respected and taken seriously. Making a disclosure may well have been difficult for her. Many women will have already encountered or may expect an unsupportive response. It is easy to make inappropriate remarks — "why don't you just leave?" — which demonstrates to the woman that the person she is speaking to has little understanding of domestic violence. By contrast, statements such as "you did not deserve to be hit" convey support. Validating the experience also entails having some understanding of how difficult it can be to leave a violent relationship, so that the woman who stays is not labeled a failure or timewaster by doctors and others.

Assessment and treatment

How detailed an assessment is undertaken will depend on the setting and context of the disclosure. It will usually be obvious whether any physical injuries need treatment and whether a detailed mental health assessment is required. Hospital referral may be necessary. Some idea of the woman's current safety and that of her children needs to be gauged in order to focus subsequent advice giving. Broadly speaking, this will entail finding out whether the woman requires a place of safety (eg a refuge), whether any children she may have are at risk and whether child protection procedures need to be followed. It is not the place of the doctor to tell her what to do, but rather to encourage and empower her to make her own decisions. Helping her with a safety plan may be something the GP can do in liaison with other agencies or members of the primary health care team and this is certainly an important area to discuss, even if only briefly, as the woman may choose not to seek help elsewhere. Advise her to keep money and important documents hidden in a safe place, as well as some clothes for herself and her children, in case she has to leave quickly. Suggest to her that she plans where she will go in the event of an emergency — this might be to friends, family or a refuge — and that she keeps useful phone numbers to hand.[10]

Domestic violence is not a diagnosis amenable to 'treatment', but referral to a counselling service (ideally one with experience of helping abused women) may be appropriate at the initial contact or at follow up. Help with drug or alcohol problems may be required at this stage or later. The input of other agencies may be crucial and the GP will need to know what local resources are available. Whether the GP makes a referral for the woman or enables the woman to refer herself will depend on what she wants. Couple counselling is generally to be avoided[11] for a number of reasons. Although violence clearly has a negative impact on a relationship, the primary problem which needs addressing is the man's violence: couple counselling may lead to the woman feeling that she is partly responsible for the violence and that she has to change in order to stop it happening. The woman may be put in more danger from the perpetrator if she is seen by him to be discussing his violence with someone else. In addition it may be a way for him to control her further — she may feel even less able to leave the relationship if he is participating in therapy with her.

Record keeping

Guidelines on care of women experiencing domestic violence emphasise the importance of keeping accurate records.[12] Evidence of violence may be requested subsequently, for example if the perpetrator is charged or sometimes to help with rehousing, although obtaining proof of physical injury should not be required for this. Injuries should be documented in as much detail as possible: body maps are recommended to illustrate injuries, although many GPs will not have these available. Photographs can be helpful and this could be suggested to the woman. GP records may also be helpful in confirming other effects of the violent situation such as mental health problems. All information should be documented clearly and the context of violent episodes recorded, particularly with regard to the perpetrator. Doctors could also suggest that the patient keep an accurate record of incidents of violence.

Information giving

As with assessment, how much information is given will depend on the context of the disclosure. The minimum that any practitioner should be able to do is to provide the woman with the phone number of the Women's Aid National Helpline (see back of report). Out of hours, the woman needs to know how to contact police, social services or Samaritans for access to a refuge. Details of local services, including the local Women's Aid group, Police Domestic Violence Unit (DVU), Victim Support, housing department and law centre may also be helpful, although these usually do not operate out of hours. The local domestic violence forum or Police Domestic Violence Unit may have useful leaflets and information guides which GPs could use.

Local information to be provided

- Branches of national organisations (eg Women's Aid)

- Police Station (Domestic Violence Unit)

- Access to emergency housing (eg District Housing Officer)

- Organisations giving legal advice and a list of solicitors

- Citizens Advice Bureau (CAB)

- Department of Social Security

- Organisations willing to help children

- Community Health Councils

- Accident and emergency departments

- Support/counselling groups

- Alcohol groups

- Organisations for specific community groups

- Organisations for men willing to receive help for their violent behaviour[13]

Follow up

GPs usually have an ongoing relationship with patients and are in a position to provide continuing support. In this respect, the care of a woman who has experienced domestic violence is similar to care for many people in difficult social situations or with chronic illness. Detailed specific and accurate information on law, housing and so on, as well as counselling may be better provided by the agencies mentioned above. The use of locally agreed guidelines could help the GP to know what services are available and from where, as well as recommending good practice generally.

With further research and knowledge about domestic violence, we can now develop the suggested four step action list into a seven step approach featuring:

- Privacy and confidentiality

- Questioning

- Respect and validation

- Assessment and treatment (medical and of the safety of the individual)

- Record keeping and concise documentation

- Information giving

- Support and follow up

The level of action will however, depend on the individual circumstances of the patient, the wishes of the patient, the ethical obligations of the doctor to maintain confidentiality, and the level of abuse and risk of serious harm.

Most disclosures in general practice will be from women who are not in a crisis situation, but continue to live in a violent relationship or have left violent relationships. Other than ensuring a minimum amount of specific information is given about help available for domestic violence, these consultations are perhaps not significantly different from work which GPs engage in every day. With some training and background knowledge they need not be excessively difficult or demanding. Understanding the resources available, both statutory and voluntary will help give a focused response.

The role of the primary health care team

With regard to identification, much of the above applies equally to other members of the primary health care team including practice nurses, health visitors and midwives. Practice nurses are increasingly involved in well-woman care and undertake new patient health checks — it may be that a disclosure will be made in these situations. Unless assessment, diagnosis or treatment at presentation clearly requires a doctor's input, then nurses are in a position to provide as much or more support and information as the GP. Health visitors may learn about the existence of domestic violence from their contacts with women and children. Midwives also need to be particularly alert for violence which may start or escalate during pregnancy, and for associated problems.

If the perpetrator is registered with the same doctor

Not uncommonly, the perpetrator will be registered with the same GP. The GP may well consider the man's behaviour towards the woman unacceptable. A discussion about domestic violence with him initiated by the GP may represent a breach of confidentiality and will rarely be possible or appropriate. It is very unlikely that a woman who has made a disclosure will wish the issue of domestic violence to be raised with her partner: fear of the perpetrator finding out is a common reason for women not revealing a history of violence. In addition many GPs would feel uncomfortable about engaging in a difficult and potentially confrontational situation with the perpetrator. However, the surgery environment can be helpful in conveying the message that domestic violence is not to be tolerated, through the display of appropriate posters and other materials. The perpetrator may be in need of medical care in the same way as any other patient and the GP has a duty to ensure that the appropriate medical care is available. On occasion, fears of violence from him towards members of the primary health care team may be justified and some attempt should be made to assess the risk to health service staff and ensure that staff are protected against such individuals. Removal of the alleged perpetrator from the doctor's list without good evidence that the patient represents a real threat to staff at the surgery, or to other patients, should be strongly discouraged.

Communication and confidentiality

Respect for confidentiality is an essential requirement for the preservation of trust between patients and health professionals. In addition to the traditional ethical obligation of medical secrecy which has been incorporated into the ethical codes of all health professionals, there is also a strong public interest in maintaining confidentiality so that individuals will be encouraged to seek appropriate treatment and share information relevant to their health and well-being. No problem arises where patients give informed consent to their information being disclosed to a third party. Nevertheless, statute, case law and professional guidance, recognises that confidentiality may be breached in exceptional cases and with appropriate justification. The GMC in its guidance *Duties of a Doctor* states:

> "*Disclosure may be necessary in the public interest where failure to disclose information may expose the patient, or others, to risk of death or serious harm. In such circumstances you should disclose information promptly to an appropriate person or authority*".[14]

Where the doctor becomes aware that a patient has been a victim of domestic abuse and is at risk of serious harm or death from a violent partner the doctor may decide, after considering all the available evidence and the wishes of the patient, to disclose this information to an appropriate third party. Where this is the case, ideally the doctor should first discuss this with the patient and explain his or her reasons for taking such action. Attempts should be made to seek the patient's approval and the doctor should ensure that the patient will not be put at increased risk if a disclosure is made. The appropriate authority will depend on the individual circumstances of the patient.

Information disclosed without consent should be the minimum necessary to achieve the objective. Health professionals who breach patients' confidentiality without consent must be prepared to justify their actions to their disciplinary bodies.

Disclosure where a child or other vulnerable person is at risk

On occasions, doctors may become aware or suspect that somebody, such as a child or other vulnerable person, living with the victim is also at risk of abuse. In this situation, the interests of that person are a paramount consideration, but the confidentiality owed to the victim cannot be disregarded. Nevertheless, knowledge or belief of abuse and neglect of a child or incapacitated adult is one exceptional circumstance which will usually justify a doctor making disclosure to an appropriate, responsible person or officer of a statutory agency. The GMC states that:

> "*If you believe a patient to be a victim of neglect or physical or sexual abuse, and unable to give or withhold consent to disclosure, you should usually give information to an appropriate responsible person or statutory authority*".[15]

Wherever possible consent to disclosure of information should be sought from the patient and from any other victims if they are capable of consenting. Disclosure of information about the alleged abuse of a competent child without his or her prior knowledge and consent could be counterproductive. It may just result in the patient withdrawing the allegation. Careful preparation is required therefore, before taking action. This issue is discussed in some detail in the BMA guideline *Confidentiality and People Under 16* which states that the duty of confidentiality owed to a person under 16 is as great as the duty owed to any other person. Nonetheless, as with adult patients there may be circumstances when a breach of confidentiality may be justified.[16]

In any situation where confidentiality is breached, the doctor must be prepared to justify his or her decision before the General Medical Council or appropriate disciplinary body. It is essential that doctors are aware of risk factors and carefully weigh up evidence obtained from a victim concerning alleged abuse of a child. It should not be assumed, for example, that simply because a violent relationship exists between the father and mother that any children are also subject to abuse. Doctors should also be aware that where the domestic abuse is disclosed by the patient in connection with the breakdown of a relationship, that allegations of abuse concerning the children may be a symptom of the acrimony and may not be able to be substantiated. On the other hand, doctors should be aware of the research into the connection between domestic violence and child abuse. Doctors may also need to consider the potential detrimental effects on a child who continuously witnesses violence in the domestic environment.

However, there comes a point after careful evaluation and reaching a critical threshold of professional concern when a doctor will consider that disclosure to a statutory agency is necessary to prevent further serious harm. It is important that the doctor refer these concerns to the statutory agencies so the appropriate multi-disciplinary discussions and planning take place, but without the fear that this will lead to an uncoordinated and/or premature action.

Sharing information with other members of the primary health care team

Increasingly, care is provided by multi-disciplinary teams and following a disclosure of domestic abuse by a patient the doctor may consider it appropriate to discuss this matter with other members of the primary health care team. The criteria governing such disclosure, as with all health information, is that the receiving health professional has a demonstrable 'need to know' a particular piece of information in the interests of patient care. The sharing of identifiable information for the convenience or interests of health workers or administrators cannot be justified.

The GMC makes it clear that where the disclosure of relevant information between health care professionals is clearly required for treatment to which a patient has agreed, the patient's explicit consent is not required. However, if the patient does not wish the doctor to share particular information with other members of the team, those wishes must be respected. It is particularly important in the context of domestic violence that the patient is involved in all stages of the decision making process, and that they retain as much control as possible over disclosures of information. They may feel threatened by the thought of others in the team knowing about their situation, and doctors may not wish to pursue the issue of sharing within a team for fear of discouraging the openness which currently exists between the doctor and the patient. All medical members of a team have a duty to make sure that other team members understand and observe confidentiality.

Doctors may obtain advice on issues of confidentiality in relation to domestic violence from the BMA Ethics department on 0171 383 6286.

---

7 Domestic violence in different health care settings

Dealing with domestic violence should be a multi-disciplinary issue for all health care professionals. Each discipline or specialty may be presented with women experiencing domestic violence in different circumstances in their lives, such as during pregnancy, and therefore each has a role to play in identifying the problem and offering support to that individual, but no one health care professional has the sole responsibility for this. It must be a collaborative approach.

Health care professionals should be open to the existence of the problem, request education and training so that they are more confident in the skilled questioning of individuals, educate themselves in the local resources and initiatives available and also accept more widely defined roles and responsibilities in the management of domestic violence.[1] Effective intervention and support early on is therefore crucial because the severity of violence has been found to escalate over time.[2]

Some professional organisations representing the various medical specialties have already issued guidelines for their members on how to identify and manage domestic violence; other professional bodies are currently preparing guidance notes. There are common elements in all of these recommendations which can be applied to all areas of medical care, but they must be tailored appropriately to the needs of the professional, the practice or setting, and the individual patient.

The Accident and Emergency Department

A decade ago domestic violence was viewed largely as a peripheral concern in accident and emergency medicine, but at the International Conference of Accident and Emergency Medicine in 1996, a session was devoted to the topic reflecting the increasing recognition of domestic violence as an important health issue.[3]

It is estimated that at some stage in their adult life, one in four women will experience domestic violence and they are highly represented among accident and emergency (A & E) department users.[4] However, it is generally accepted that at present the specialty is failing these women. This is due to many factors, including an increase in the number of attending patients at accident and emergency departments, increasing throughput, shortages of staff, pressures on resources and time, and the attitudes of the staff themselves towards domestic violence. All of this leads to a lower rate of identification of women experiencing domestic violence, poor documentation of those that have been identified, and poor attitudes of staff and inter-agency co-ordination.[5]

"Often the presenting complaint is only half of the picture"

There is a belief amongst accident and emergency staff that because of the high turnover of patients and the constraints mentioned above, their intervention has little effect with the patient often returning to an abusive relationship to be hurt again. Access to follow-up information and longer term progress of the patients is generally not available to reinforce the utility of the intervention. However, Stevens (1997) states, the nature of domestic violence itself means that health professionals assist in a process of empowerment and self-management by the woman of her situation, and that it may be some considerable time before she reaches the point in that process where she is ready to take definitive action. Thus it must be reinforced that an apparently unsuccessful interaction with an abused patient may, firstly, have been more successful than supposed, and secondly, that it is not a reason to withhold support from the next patient.[6]

Studies have shown that if routine screening for abuse were to take place at the A & E stage, the rates of identification would increase significantly. Norton *et al* (1995) found that if patients had the five-question Abuse Assessment Screen added to the standard social services interview, the lifetime prevalence rate identified rose from 4% to 41% and the incidence of recent abuse from 3% to 15%.[7] McLeer and Anwar (1989) found that the introduction of a screening protocol raised the detection rate of domestic violence from 5.6% to 30%. However, when they revisited the department eight years later, the staff had become complacent about the protocol and the detection rate had dropped to 7.7%. Further research into the efficacy of screening in UK health care settings is required to determine a practice that is both acceptable to women and doctors and is sensitive to different cultures and areas.

Thus staff education is vital in sustaining a successful domestic violence identification programme.[8] A study by Helton *et al* (1987) showed that after an educational programme, health care professionals were far more willing to assess and intervene with battered, pregnant women.[9] Another study by Bokunewicz and Copel (1992) showed that emergency nurses had changed their attitudes after a 60 minute presentation on the cycle of violence theory.[10]

Successful domestic violence protocols must be able to be practically implemented with an accident and emergency department operating within all of the usual constraints of time, resources, patient numbers and staff. The staff must also believe in the utility of their interventions and must be continually educated and encouraged to incorporate the protocol into their normal routines.

Stevens (1997) concludes that a successful domestic violence protocol that works within the above parameters is likely to consist of brief screening by the A & E staff, who hand over to a dedicated domestic violence team member who in turn acts as the survivor's advocate and link to the community and hospital services. The protocol must be planned and funded to be consistently deliverable around the clock, every day of the year and it must be backed by an educational programme, preferably taught by members of a dedicated domestic violence team.[11] In reality, the likelihood of a dedicated team would require a definite initiative from the local Health Authority.

In 1994, guidelines on domestic violence were issued to every A & E department in the UK.[12] They recommended the following:

- the attending staff be thorough in their examination of injuries and remember that often the presenting complaint is only part of the picture;

- document the injuries meticulously;

- treat the injuries that are presented;

- approach the patient and ask direct questions gently about her injuries and encourage the patient's right to make her own decisions;

- discuss the next steps for the patient and offer contact numbers and written information where available and helpful.

There is a clear need to monitor the prevalence, identification and referral procedures in A & E departments. Safety audits which assess things such as the safety of A & E premises, and the safety of methods of working with individuals affected by domestic violence, should be included in medical audits. Clear guidance is also needed on what inter-agency working entails, and on what the responsibilities of A & E staff are to work in an inter-agency way. In view of the growing awareness of the links between domestic violence and child probation issues, specific guidance is needed for A & E staff on child protection responsibilities in the context of domestic violence.

Obstetrics and Gynaecology

Research provides overwhelming evidence that domestic violence may begin or escalate in pregnancy.[13,14] The risk of moderate to severe violence appears to be greatest in the postpartum period.[15] Domestic violence can lead to physical and psychological harm of the mother and baby and is associated with adverse pregnancy outcomes such as miscarriage, still birth and preterm labour.[16]

As the obstetrician is the key health professional in contact with women with, or at high risk of, complications in their pregnancy, then the obstetrician is in an important position to identify any incidents of domestic violence. Persistent gynaecological complaints can also be important presentations of domestic violence and so the gynaecologist also has a very important role to play.

"*Domestic violence often starts or escalates in pregnancy***"**

To encourage the disclosure of sensitive information, all pregnant women should have at least one consultation with the lead professional involved in her pregnancy care which is not attended by the partner or any family member, and that a set of confidential notes should be kept separate from those held by the patient. Where domestic violence is disclosed, the doctor should be non-judgmental and offer confidential support and information about the appropriate agencies that may be able to help. The Royal College of Obstetricians and Gynaecologists (RCOG) report (1997) advises obstetricians to respect patients' confidentiality and to seek consent before sharing information about acts of violence. Consent may not be needed in some circumstances, if the health professional feels that the health or safety of the patient is at real risk. In the latter instance especially, the nature of, and reasons for, disclosure must be clearly documented.[17]

Education and training to increase doctors' awareness of skills in recognising and identifying women suspected of experiencing domestic violence is needed. In 1995, in a study of 6568 obstetricians/gynaecologists, a lack of education was identified as the most common barrier the doctors had to questioning for domestic violence. The feeling that abuse was not a problem in their patients (46%), lack of time to deal with abuse (39.2%), and frustration that the doctor cannot help the individual (34.2%) were other common barriers.[18] Other research has also shown that the training and education of health professionals in increasing their knowledge and willingness to identify domestic violence thus increase rates of detection.[19,20] A study group of the RCOG has recommended that teaching about domestic violence should be an integral part of training for obstetricians and gynaecologists, and their ability to address this delicate issue should be evaluated in examinations.[21] This is to be welcomed.

Psychiatry

As well as physical injury, domestic violence can have serious psychological effects such as anxiety, depression, suicide and post traumatic stress disorder. Studies have shown that women experiencing domestic violence comprise a large proportion of those referred to the psychiatric emergency service, or institutionalised in psychiatric facilities.[22,23]

A strong association has also been found between domestic violence and psychiatric illness, parasuicide, alcohol and drug abuse.[24] Roberts *et al* (1997) found that in a study conducted in 1991 of victims of domestic violence attendees in an emergency department, there was a progression from multiple attendances in the emergency department for physical trauma over five years, to alcohol and drug problems, to current violence and suicide attempts.[25]

Psychiatrists' roles in dealing with domestic violence lie in early diagnosis and support, as most individuals will not readily admit to the abuse. Knowledge of significant indicators can facilitate the identification of women who have experienced abuse and lead to the development of more effective identification.[26] Understanding the psychology of both the perpetrator and the victim will also be helpful. There is no single treatment for domestic violence, instead the psychiatrist must support the woman through a process of empowerment so that she will eventually make a decision herself. Psychiatrists may be able to offer particular support services such as stress clinics and perpetrators' projects. Unfortunately, few guidelines exist at present that offer help to psychiatrists in increasing identification and management of domestic violence cases. Raising awareness of the presentations and manifestations of domestic violence in psychiatric conditions is of paramount importance as some will be more obvious than others. Education and training is essential in achieving this aim.

Nursing

Nurses are often in a unique position to identify abuse, but despite this and the evidence that domestic violence signifies a huge social and health problem, it remains a low-key issue in nursing at present.[27] The reasons for this are similar to any other of the specialities discussed; lack of understanding of the issue; lack of a protocol once abuse is disclosed;

lack of education and training, which all leads to a lack of confidence about how to intervene in possible cases of disclosure.

Nurses work in a variety of health and community settings and may often be the first people, outside of the family, to know that abuse is occurring. Understanding the varied contexts of nursing is important. For example, nurses working in accident and emergency settings are more likely to be involved with acute incidents. School nurses may be well placed to work with children on violence prevention. Indeed, projects on violence prevention which have closely worked with school nurses have already been developed in Islington, Greenwich and, more recently, East Surrey. Community health care teams (health visitors, community paediatric and midwifery services etc) have by the nature of their role, greater access to, and involvement in, a woman's world and may develop more empathy and understanding of the difficulties and fears which a woman has to cope with in her daily efforts to manage her life and that of her children.[28] Community care nurses should also be aware of abuse within the home care context. Practice nurses and health visitors are also likely to come into contact with women experiencing domestic violence. Mezey *et al* (1998) found that women attending GP's surgeries were more likely to disclose domestic violence to their health visitor, although it is unclear whether this was related to the fact that health visitors were more likely to be female, or to their different approaches to women.[29]

Nurses in all settings and contexts need to receive training to improve their awareness of domestic violence and become involved in drawing up good practice guidelines in this area as soon as possible. The Royal College of Nursing (RCN) have convened a working party to consider the issue of domestic violence and the role of the nurse in dealing with it. They are due to publish their findings towards the end of 1998 which are expected to offer guidance on how to identify and manage domestic violence through, for example, education and training initiatives and knowledge of local resources.

Midwifery

As discussed previously, most research has found that violence may begin or escalate in pregnancy,[30] and that violence can be associated with adverse pregnancy outcomes such as miscarriage, still birth and preterm labour.[31]

Since the main role of the midwife is to care for and ensure the health and safety of both mother and baby, the midwife appears to be well placed to have a greater role in identifying and discussing domestic violence.

In response to a rising number of enquiries from midwives about domestic violence, the Royal College of Midwives (RCM) issued a set of guidelines in 1997 for safe and appropriate midwifery practice in dealing with domestic violence. The RCM believes that midwives are ideally placed to identify abused women and that every midwife should assume a role in the detection and management of this. They state that domestic violence in pregnancy is best challenged by a multi-disciplinary approach, but this is often hampered by an inadequate co-ordination of services.[32]

The College recommends that a systematic and structured framework should be developed to facilitate the role of the midwife by introducing policies and guidelines within maternity units. To help in achieving this, the guidelines detail a number of clinical, psychological and social indicators which can alert a midwife to the possibility of potential or actual abuse and offers a specific step-by-step action list concerning identification questions, documentation of abuse and responding to disclosure of abuse. Studies have shown that the use of structured screening questions such as those suggested by the RCM can significantly improve detection rates of domestic violence.[33,34] The RCM guidelines state that all midwives should be aware of the services and resources available in their local area so that once domestic violence has been disclosed, the midwife can provide a response, supplying the woman with helpful information, a referral to an appropriate agency, or any other action deemed necessary.

Domestic violence is a significant factor in maternal and perinatal mortality and morbidity. Although many midwives may already suspect domestic violence, in the absence of a referral process they are often unsure of what action to take or advice to offer. Midwives need guidelines at local levels to support intervention. Such guidelines should not be prescriptive or mandatory, but should offer an inter-disciplinary approach which does not leave the responsibility of the woman experiencing violence to the one professional group or individual. Advice should also be offered on the local organisations and agencies available in the local community.[35] Midwives are ideally placed to identify abuse and their role should be included in a collaborative approach to addressing domestic violence.

> **❝All doctors at some point in their professional lives are likely to come into contact with patients who have experienced domestic violence❞**

This list of health care professionals is by no means exhaustive. Orthopaedists, paediatricians, ear, nose and throat specialists as well as dentists and all other health care professionals have a crucial role to play in the identification and management of domestic violence. It must be remembered that all doctors at some point in their professional lives are likely to come into contact with patients who are experiencing, or who have experienced, domestic violence. In all health care settings where domestic violence may be disclosed, whether it is physical injury or psychological harm, the seven-step action list should be followed immediately to provide a basic and standard level of care and support to those individuals.

8 Adopting an inter-agency approach

Inter-agency working

The promotion of inter-agency working has become an important part of government policy on domestic violence in the 1990s. There has been a considerable expansion of these inter-agency initiatives across the UK and some have brought substantial improvements in service delivery.[1] Health care professionals have played a small part in these developments[2] although there are exceptions where health authorities have taken a lead role.[3]

There is no set model for inter-agency working, although all share the broad common aim of drawing together a range of agencies to tackle domestic violence in a more coordinated way. How the various initiatives operate and what they do varies from area to area.[4] The inter-agency approach has been dominated by the 'forum method' of working where representatives from local agencies gather together, in formal or informal meetings, to share information and coordinate a range of activities from training to policy development to service provision. More than 150 inter-agency fora on domestic violence exist throughout the UK and bring together a wide range of statutory and voluntary sector agencies.[5] GPs and health care workers may feel that they have little to offer or to gain from this forum method, possibly because of issues of individual patient confidentiality, and research from the USA shows some resistance amongst doctors to this style of working.[6] The very real difficulties that GPs face in becoming involved with inter-agency work on domestic violence should also be considered. Most meeting times which are convenient for other agencies tend to coincide with GP surgery times making it difficult for GPs to attend. If they do take time away from the practice, then locum cover for the care of their patients is also required which means that the GP incurs a personal cost in attending meetings. The Home Office Circular on inter-agency working issued in 1995 emphasised the benefits to be gained through the coordination of services working in local communities.[7] The new proposals for the NHS emphasise closer working between social services, community groups and health care providers at the local level in Primary Care Groups.[8] As yet there has been little guidance for GPs and other health care professionals on their roles and responsibilities regarding inter-agency working. Guidelines on this would be particularly welcome and might help to break down some of the barriers to participation. Apparent lack of participation at present suggests to other more active agencies that the medical profession has yet to take domestic violence seriously.

Inter-agency initiatives on domestic violence have a great deal to offer GPs and health service providers, particularly in terms of training opportunities, information on support groups, resources and referral agencies, guidance on policy and best practice, including anti-discriminatory methods of working. If GPs and health care professionals do start to ask patients about domestic violence, some work with, and knowledge of, the responsibilities of other agencies will be necessary so that appropriate referrals can be made. Fora can usually be contacted through the local police or through the domestic violence unit.

Legal advice

Enabling people who experience domestic violence to gain an understanding of the services available to them is a crucial part of safety planning. Legal advice on domestic violence matters is available from local solicitors, the Citizens Advice Bureau (CAB), Women's Aid refuges and the helpline services listed in the appendix to this report. It is recommended that primary health care teams should hold a brief, up to date contact list for referral purposes. In areas where there are inter-agency fora, this information is easily obtained.

Involving the police

An earlier section of this report considered whether or not a doctor should disclose information to the police. Women may be reluctant to involve the police for a number of reasons. For instance, they may not see any benefits to be gained from involving them or pursuing a case through to prosecution.[9] There has been some debate over the degree to which the police should use their powers to compel those who have experienced domestic violence to give evidence for the prosecution of abusive partners.[10] If the police are called, the woman's main motive is often to stop the violence, rather than to prosecute her partner. Women from ethnic minorities and women with insecure immigration status may be especially reluctant to involve the police.[11,12] Women may also be fearful that if the police become involved then social services will be notified and they may risk 'losing' their children. This is likely to be a particular concern for women in the health care setting because doctors have knowledge of her vulnerabilities.

If the police are called to a domestic violence incident, their main responsibility is to protect the victim and any children from further violence and to arrest the assailant if there has been an offence. The Home Office Circular issued to the police in 1990[13] recommended that the police adopt a more interventionist stance by arresting assailants when an offence has been committed, recording and investigating incidents of domestic violence in the same way as other assaults, and offering protection and support to victims. The circular also urged police forces to set up dedicated units, with specialist staff, to work with domestic violence cases, and to liaise between the police and other agencies in local communities. Many police force areas now have Domestic Violence Units (DVU) with staff who work full time (usually 9 to 5 office hours) only on domestic violence issues. Officers from DVUs have often taken a lead role in setting up forums and coordinating inter-agency working.[14] They can be a very good starting point for information and guidance on domestic violence issues for GPs and primary health care teams.

The Home Office guidance to the police suggests that in all domestic violence cases the police should:

- respond quickly;

- separate the parties to the dispute and talk to them separately;

- arrest the offender if there is evidence of an assault or other offence (such as a breach of bail or an injunction);

- arrange for emergency medical treatment;

- have a woman officer present if available;

- give information on other sources of help available, eg from Women's Aid refuges (some forces issue small *aide memoire* cards to officers for this purpose);

- provide transport to a refuge or other safe place;

- provide protection while collecting any belongings from the home;

- keep a record of all reported incidents of domestic violence and refer to specialist domestic violence officers, where available;

- provide information on the action taken including forthcoming court dates and bail release dates.

Offences for which the police can arrest (arrestable offences) include common assault (pushing, hitting, threats etc which lead to minor bruising, scratches, grazes, a black eye etc); an assault occasioning actual bodily harm (such as shock, multiple bruising, cuts, minor fractures); grievous bodily harm (where a serious injury was intended or resulted); rape, attempted rape, indecent assault, attempted murder and murder; criminal damage to property; criminal harassment as defined under the Protection From Harassment Act 1997.

The police can also arrest someone who breaks bail conditions or who breaches an injunction which includes powers of arrest. If there are no statutory powers of arrest the police may also arrest the offender if he has caused a 'breach of the peace'. Once arrested, the police can hold the offender before charging him for up to 24 hours.[15] This can give the woman time to seek further advice, to consider her options and to find a place of safety.

The police response to domestic violence has changed substantially in recent years, although not all the changes in policy and thinking have affected the work of uniformed officers working in the community and practice still varies from area to area.[16] Officers have discretion about whether or not to arrest, caution or to take other action to intervene following a call relating to a domestic violence incident. In 1997, the HM Inspectorate of Constabulary in Scotland published a report on the police responses to women experiencing domestic violence. The report considered how domestic violence was being addressed by the police force and to help identify areas of good practice and develop strategies to further improve the police response.[17]

Court Orders for personal protection and occupation of the home

Adults who experience domestic violence can apply to the magistrates (family proceedings courts) or to a county court for an order which prohibits any further violence or 'molestation' and, in some cases, for an order regulating occupation of the family home. Children can now apply, with leave of the court, for similar orders from the High Court. Part IV of the Family Law Act came into force on 1 October 1997. This provides for new, broader non-molestation orders and occupation orders to be made by the courts. Non-molestation orders prevent the perpetrator from molesting the partner and/or any relevant child. Occupation orders can regulate occupation of the home by permitting a person who has been thrown out of the home re-entry or by excluding the perpetrator from the home, temporarily or for a longer period of time.

Key changes introduced by the new law include:

- a wider range of people can get orders to protect them from domestic violence — including children, people who have not recently or who have never cohabited with their partners, lesbian and gay people affected by domestic violence from partners;

- most orders are likely to carry powers of arrest;

- occupation orders now range from short term orders to orders of longer duration, so the courts can provide protection and security which goes beyond a 'first aid' approach;

- the time period for which many orders were previously available has increased to a period of six months;

- occupation orders may now be granted *ex parte* (in the absence of the perpetrator from the court);

- powers of arrest may be attached to *ex parte* occupation orders.

Remedies under the new law are available to 'associated persons'. Under S62(4) and (5) of the 1996 Family Law Act these are:

- persons who are or who have been married to one another;

- cohabitants or former cohabitants;

- persons who live or who have lived in the same household (other than by reason of one of them being the other's employee, tenant, lodger or boarder);

- certain relatives — parents/stepparents, children/stepchildren, grandparents, grandchildren, brothers, sisters, uncles, aunts, nieces, nephews of a person against whom the order is sought or of that person's spouse or former spouse;

- people who have agreed to marry one another;

- in relation to a child, parents or people who have parental responsibility for the child;

- a natural parent or grandparent of a child freed for adoption where the other is either the adoptive parent, a person who has applied for adoption, or the child who has been adopted or freed for adoption;

- persons who are parties to the same family proceedings.

Molestation orders can also now be made to protect lesbian or gay people from a partner's violence if they are living, or have lived, in the same household.

'Molestation' is not defined in the Act but on the basis of previous cases which have passed through the courts, this refers to any conduct which could be regarded as being harassment, intimidation or pestering. In deciding whether to exercise its powers to make a non-molestation order the court shall have regard to all the circumstances of the case

67

including the need to secure the health, safety and well being of the applicant and any relevant child (S42(5)).

Various occupation orders are available (Ss33 to 41). The type of order available will vary if the person applying has some right or entitlement to occupy (ie she has tenancy rights or matrimonial rights to occupy). Provisions are made in the Act for spouses, former spouses, cohabitants and former cohabitants who have no rights to occupy, in relation to partners/ex partners who have, or who also lack, occupation rights, but these are of limited duration — six months in the first instance.

If a person has an entitlement to occupy the court considers applications for occupation orders with regard to all the circumstances, in particular:

- the housing needs and resources of the parties and children;

- the parties' financial resources;

- the likely effect of the order (or lack of one) on the health, safety and well being of the parties or any relevant child;

- the conduct of the parties.

A 'balance of harm test' is also applied. This means that the court should make an order if it is likely that the applicant or a relevant child will suffer harm attributable to the respondent's conduct if no order is made. This is unless it appears to the court that the respondent and a relevant child will suffer harm if an order is made, or that this harm is likely to be as great as or greater than the harm to the applicant or child if no order is made (S33(7)).

For married or once married persons who lack occupation rights, the court will in addition consider:

- the length of time which has elapsed since the parties stopped living together;

- the length of time since a divorce or annulment;

- the existence of any current legal proceedings.

For cohabitants and former cohabitants who lack rights to occupy, the court will in addition consider:

- the nature of the relationship;

- whether or not there are any children;

- the duration of cohabitation;

- the length of time which has elapsed since they stopped living together;

● the existence of any current legal proceedings.

Medical issues and the Family Law Act 1996

There has been no research in the UK on the nature of and the degree of the involvement of the medical profession in domestic violence cases before the courts. It is therefore difficult to assess the likely impact of the new law; future monitoring would be worthwhile. The Act is littered with references to health, so it is likely GPs may be asked more frequently to provide medical evidence to support applications for non-molestation or occupation orders, particularly if orders are applied for *ex parte*. The introduction of the 'balance of harm test' may mean that the need for medical evidence to support injunction applications will increase. Accurate records should be kept of any injuries and of any harm or impairment of a woman's or to a child's health as a result of the domestic violence. Training for doctors on recording injuries for evidential purposes is recommended.

Section 48(4) of the 1996 Act may raise some major issues for the medical profession. This gives the civil court powers similar to those available to the Crown Court under the Mental Health Act 1983 S35. Courts can now remand a person arrested for domestic violence for up to four weeks to enable a medical report to be made, if there is reason to suspect that the person is suffering from mental illness or a severe mental impairment. A hospital order may subsequently be made. The extent to which these provisions will be used remains to be seen. Monitoring may be needed because an increased use might raise civil liberties concerns and would have an impact upon mental health services.

Protection from Harassment Act 1997

The Protection from Harassment Act 1997 came into effect on 16 June 1997. There is some overlap between the provisions covered by this Act and those contained within Part IV of the Family Law Act which came into force on 1 October 1997. The Protection from Harassment Act aims to tackle the problem of 'stalking' and harassment which may affect people in the public eye, but also (as the earlier section of this report shows) commonly affects women leaving a violent partner. The law provides for both civil and criminal law remedies against 'stalking' and harassment. The 1997 Act created two new criminal offences:

● Criminal harassment (S2), a summary offence tried in the magistrates courts;

● An offence involving fear of violence (S4), tried by magistrates or as an indictable offence in the Crown Court. An offence is committed if a person, on at least two occasions, is caused to fear that violence will be used against them and the person causing the fear knew this would be the result of his behaviour.

Harassment means the offender has been pursuing a 'course of conduct' (conduct on at least two occasions) which they know, or ought to know, amounts to harassment of the other person. A 'reasonable person' test is applied to assess whether or not the course of conduct amounts to harassment, ie the court considers whether or not a (hypothetical) reasonable person possessing the same information would consider the course of conduct to be harassment. Conduct is taken to include speech.

Harassment under S2 is an arrestable offence. If a person is found guilty under S4, of causing another fear of violence, they may be imprisoned for up to five years. A court may also make a restraining order against a person convicted of harassment. Breach of this order will also be a criminal offence.

The 1997 Act also created additional civil law remedies to deal with harassment. S3 of the Act provides for damages to be claimed for the anxiety caused by, or any financial loss resulting from the offender's harassment. Courts can make interlocutory and final injunction orders if there is a claim for damages.

The 1997 Act may make it easier for women to get legal protection from partners or ex partners who subject them to harassment and behaviour which stops short of 'violence' but nonetheless causes fear. Courts may be more likely to look at the cumulative impact of the behaviour. The impact which the new provisions have will depend largely upon the police response. There are no provisions in the Act to attach powers of arrest to an order and currently there appear to be no provisions in force for courts to issue arrest warrants.

Medical issues and Part IV of the Family Law Act 1997

As with Part IV of the Family Law Act, the Protection from Harassment Act 1997 may mean that GPs will be asked to provide medical evidence to support applications. The same comments apply as regards keeping accurate records of any injuries and of any harm or impairment of a woman's or to a child's health as a result of the domestic violence (see previous section on GP record keeping, p48). Evidence of a pattern of conduct over time may be needed.

It can be noted that only the Protection from Harassment Act 1997 offers protection to individuals against non-physical forms of domestic violence, yet we know that physical violence is only one aspect of continued domestic violence. This lack of protection in the law is a major concern, although it can be appreciated that non-physical violence is more difficult to quantify and prove.

Child protection and domestic violence

General practitioners and other members of the primary health care team have an important role to play in the prevention, identification and subsequent management of child abuse. The policy and legislative framework governing the inter-agency approach to child protection issues is set out in the Children Act 1989, in Department of Health guidance[18] and often at the local level in child protection manuals and guidelines. The links between domestic violence to the mother and abuse of the child are increasingly being acknowledged by child protection agencies and many of the local child protection manuals and guidelines now offer guidance on this matter.[19] The child's welfare is the 'paramount issue' of concern in child protection matters. An earlier section in this report has shown that providing support and protection to the mother is increasingly being recommended as a most effective child protective strategy where there is domestic violence.

Recent amendments to the Children Act may make it easier to protect children and mothers from domestic violence. Schedule 6 of the Family Law Act 1996 amended S38A(1) of the Children Act 1989 to enable courts to oust child abusers from the home in order to protect the children. The power to oust the abuser is linked to applications for interim care orders or to applications for emergency protection orders. Abusers can be excluded if there is reasonable cause to believe that the child would cease to — or would be likely to cease to — suffer significant harm as a result. The exclusion can only be made if a suitable carer remains in the home, who is willing and able to care for the child, and they consent to the exclusion. Courts may attach powers of arrest to these exclusion orders. The new provisions may mean that women who experience domestic violence will be less fearful of 'losing' their children if they become involved with social services. The amendment means that social services, rather than the woman herself, will have the responsibility to organise legal proceedings to oust the abuser.

Services for children living through domestic violence

Up until relatively recently, the needs of children affected by domestic violence have been ignored by most of the relevant service providers, apart from within Women's refuges.[20] Refuges have developed expertise in providing emotional and practical support for children, from counselling to play therapy, to practical guidance on safety planning and self protection. It is recommended that health care providers develop and maintain good inter-agency working relationships with local refuge groups. Other agencies which may offer support to children in the local community include:

- the child guidance service;

- NSPCC, NCH Action For Children, Barnados projects;

- the local authority social services department;

- In many parts of the country contact centres offer a venue for children who have difficulties with parental contact arrangements. Centres can usually be contacted through the Family Court Welfare service.

Emergency accommodation and housing

Women's Aid refuges offer safe accommodation, practical support, advice and after care to women and children who experience domestic violence. Most refuges can be contacted out of office hours, either by telephoning a special helpline number or via the police, through social services or, in some areas, through groups such as the Samaritans. There are a more limited number of refuges which cater specifically for the needs of black and ethnic minority women and for women with learning disabilities. Many refuges try to cater for the needs of women and children with disabilities, but suitable accommodation is severely limited. It is particularly difficult for refuges to accommodate women with special needs, with drug or alcohol problems, and finding a place of safety for women with these difficulties can be hard. This lack of provision will inevitably have an impact on the health of women and children with special needs and disabilities.

Women who want help with housing issues, but who do not want to move into a refuge can approach the local housing department for advice, and in some cases temporary accommodation. The Housing Act 1996 now sets out the responsibilities of housing departments as regards homeless persons, including people made homeless as a result of domestic violence from an 'associated person'. Housing authorities are not required to offer permanent accommodation to homeless persons under the Act, although they may provide temporary accommodation for up to two years. Whether or not a person might be eligible for temporary accommodation depends on the result of enquiries made to establish:

- whether the applicant is homeless or threatened with homelessness;

- the eligibility for assistance ('persons from abroad' are defined as having less eligibility);

- priority need (this includes people with children, pregnant women, people who are vulnerable due to ill health, old age, mental or physical ability, or who are made homeless because of an emergency such as a fire or flood);

- whether the applicant is intentionally homeless (whether they did something or failed to do something which resulted in the loss of, or failure to take up accommodation);

- whether the applicant has a local connection with the area via residence, family or employment ties.

There is a shortage of affordable, safe and secure housing for women and children fleeing domestic violence.[21] Insecure housing, moving from one shorthold tenancy to another, will inevitably have an impact upon the health and welfare of women and children. There is a need for research which explores the health and social impact which the new legislation has upon people affected by domestic violence.

Help for perpetrators

In many parts of the country, the probation service and voluntary sector have developed groups which work with perpetrators to challenge and change violent behaviour. There is great variation in the form and function of perpetrator groups and some may be rather a mixed blessing for the perpetrator's partner. Perpetrator projects which are viewed as a 'soft option' or which provide couple counselling or anger management are generally viewed as being unhelpful in the context of domestic violence.[22] Projects which have drawn upon the Duluth re-educative approach, which also provide support and attempt to monitor the safety of partners have been established in the UK, and have recently been evaluated favourably in comparison to traditional criminal justice interventions by themselves.[23,24] Men's programmes vary also in the way in which referrals are channelled. Some projects welcome self referrals whilst others require referral via the courts or probation service. The local probation service, domestic violence forum, refuge or police domestic violence unit are a good source for further information on local groups for perpetrators. However, the success of a referral to such a group will be minimal if the perpetrator is not able to accept that he has a problem.

9 Conclusions and recommendations

Conclusions

Domestic violence is a considerable medical and social issue. It affects a significant proportion of the population at some time during their lives, although research has not yet shown precisely how frequent or repeated it is. Domestic violence is a serious crime which has a substantial impact upon the health and welfare of adults and children. Approximately one in four women will experience domestic violence at some stage in their life and of these around only 25% of all incidents are reported to the police.[1] 69% of domestic violence incidents are likely to result in injury which is more than any other violent crime.[2] It is usually repeated over many years and can escalate and intensify. It is estimated that approximately only 30% of women seek help soon after the first or subsequent attack.[3]

It is known that many women who experience domestic violence go undetected in health care settings, and the limited evidence for this lack of identification comes both from doctors and from women themselves. Reasons advocated for women not reporting domestic violence have been outlined earlier (see Chapter Two). Reasons why doctors largely do not identify women who have experienced domestic violence have also been advocated and include:

- doctors' fears or experiences of exploring the issues of domestic violence;
- lack of knowledge of community resources;
- fear of offending the woman and jeopardising the doctor-patient relationship;
- lack of time;
- lack of training;
- lack of control;
- infrequent patient visits;
- unresponsiveness of patients to questions;
- feeling powerless; not being able to fix the situation.

The health and social costs and consequences of domestic violence are extensive and have been detailed in Chapter Four of this report. There are a wide variety of manifestations and presentations of domestic violence, ranging from various non-specific symptoms and signs, such as insomnia and anxiety, to more specific presentations due to acts of violence against women, such as injury to the breasts. Depression, drug and alcohol abuse and other mental health problems are also associated with, and may be exacerbated by, domestic violence. Domestic violence significantly affects the mental and physical health of large numbers of women and their children and, therefore, doctors and other health professionals are inevitably involved in providing care for this group.

It has been argued that domestic violence to men by women occurs as frequently as domestic violence by men against women, but there is at present little evidence and research data to support this claim. There may be many reasons why men are more likely not to disclose domestic violence, including the man's feelings of shame, stigma and of not being taken seriously.[1] The circumstances of male reported domestic violence are also not known, for example, if the perpetrator was a male or whether the woman acted in self defence. Detailed research is therefore required to consider both the prevalence of male reported domestic violence and also the circumstances in which it occurs.

It must always be remembered that disclosures of violence require confidentiality, privacy, sensitive questioning and a non-judgmental attitude. Questioning is essential and unless asked directly, women may not disclose violence.

Identification of individuals experiencing domestic violence is the first step towards ensuring appropriate care, and the following action list should be followed by all health care professionals to ensure a basic standard level of care to all individuals.

Action list for health care professionals
● Privacy and confidentiality
● Questioning
● Respect and validation
● Assessment and treatment
● Record keeping and concise documentation
● Information giving
● Support and follow up

The annual report of the Chief Medical Officer for England and Wales, *On the State of the Public Health 1996*, states that effective implementation of the new legislation in Part IV of the Family Law Act will require improved recognition of domestic violence, further facilities to help, advise and support women who experience domestic violence, and an effective interface with other agencies, especially social services and the criminal justice system.[5] With the recent publications of the Green Papers[6,7] and the White Papers[8,9] there appears to be scope for the NHS to make great strides in the development of practice in relation to patients who experience domestic violence. The Primary Care Groups and Health Improvement Programmes suggested by the White Papers may provide more opportunity for a policy on change and management referral for inter-agency co-ordination initiatives. Directors of Public Health and Health Authorities could all work towards addressing this problem. We applaud the mention of domestic violence in the Scottish Green Paper,[10] but regret the lack of any mention in the England and Wales equivalent.[11] The Green Papers do propose that long term service agreements will replace annual contracts which will have explicit quality standards. It should therefore be recommended that long term service agreements make explicit reference to the quality and accessibility of services for people who experience domestic violence.

Until recently health care professionals have not fully considered the challenges which domestic violence raises. There is a need for the medical profession to take a more pro-active approach and to do this at all levels of organisational responsibility.

Health care professionals should recognise that they are responsible for managing violence against women and that they can make a difference. This could be at any episode in a woman's life and for various presentations that may often not seem related. It is important for the health care professional to realise, however, that this is not a sole responsibility, and must be part of a multi-disciplinary and inter-agency approach. The medical profession can also learn from organisations such as the Women's Aid Federation that are presently far ahead of the medical profession in dealing with domestic violence. In health care settings, domestic violence is under-researched and there is little good research that has been done looking at the efficacy of interventions in dealing with domestic violence. What research exists is often not of high quality and is therefore not evidence based in the way that much medical research is today. This does not mean that domestic violence should be dismissed as a health care issue, but that much greater input is needed. Lack of evidence does not equate with evidence against a particular way of behaving.

> **❝*Health professionals assist in a process of empowerment and self-management by the woman of her situation, and it may be some time before she is ready to take definitive action*❞**

Intervention by the doctor is not just directly trying to stop the violence, but includes validation of the violence, medical treatment, information giving and support, and facilitating referral. Treatment of symptoms of domestic violence, whether psychiatric or physical, are unlikely to be more than palliative, as long as the patient remains in a high risk situation. Stevens (1997) states that the nature of domestic violence itself means that health professionals assist in a process of empowerment and self-management by the woman of her situation, and that it may be some considerable time before she reaches the point where she is ready to take definitive action. Thus it must be reinforced that an apparently unsuccessful interaction with an abused patient may have been more successful than supposed. Professionals who are able to develop their knowledge and understanding of domestic violence and its impact upon women and children will be in a better position both to protect children and provide appropriate support to parents. However, inter-agency guidelines, policy and practice guidelines are ineffective by themselves. Their implementation will be limited unless there are good monitoring procedures.[12]

Few guidelines for health professionals on domestic violence have been produced, although the Royal College of Obstetricians and Gynaecologists recently published their report on *Violence Against Women*[13] which considered domestic violence, and detailed in particular the role of the obstetrician and gynaecologist. As the major professional organisation representing all doctors in the UK, the British Medical Association (BMA) through this report aims to lead the way in encouraging all health professionals in all disciplines to raise their awareness of the problem of domestic violence, and to develop strategies to identify and reduce the injuries caused.

Recommendations

National policies

1   The BMA welcomes the statement of the Chief Medical Officer for England and Wales in his annual report *On the State of the Public Health 1996*, confirming that the Department of Health will help to ensure that connections are made between various existing initiatives; to assist where appropriate in informing health care professionals about the nature and extent of the problem, and to co-ordinate effective use of NHS resources in helping those subject to domestic violence. The BMA urges that this is made a priority and should include an increased provision of funding and resources.

2   The Departments of Health for England and Wales and Scotland through their White and Green Papers should develop inter-agency strategies in dealing with domestic violence. This could be included in the remit of the newly created primary care groups and health improvement programmes.

3   Identification and management of these problems are important components of the 'Health Improvement Programmes' which are the responsibility of health authorities under the new White Papers. It should be a requirement of all health authorities that health improvement programmes contain inter-agency agreements to provide for the recognition and management of domestic violence. There should be continuous monitoring of the frequency of its occurrence and of the effectiveness of the solutions available.

4   The development and provision of social and legal services that could offer support and help to those experiencing domestic violence should be encouraged. Local authorities could assist in funding refuges, raising public awareness, assisting in the provision of a helpline, improved access to safe housing and improved provision of legal advice and protection.

5   Service providers should have an understanding of the nature, context and pattern of domestic violence for the provision of services to both men and women. Services should be 'needs-led' which would enable providers to be accountable to service users.

6   Police records, criminal statistics and government crime surveys all tend to undercount domestic violence because they use a narrower definition of domestic violence which is based upon acts of criminal, physical violence occurring within a limited period of time, usually within the past 12 months. Amendments should be made to the laws on violence and harassment so that protection and support can be

offered for non-physical aspects of domestic violence also. The identification of abuse at three levels such as in the Hackney study could be adopted, ie:

- Type A abuse = non-physical, verbal, financial or psychological

- Type B abuse = physical abuse such as slaps and punches

- Type C abuse = physical and sexual abuse which is likely to require medical attention, such as kicks in the face, attempted strangulation etc.

The medical profession

7   Increased awareness of the existence of domestic violence is urgently required by all health professionals. Professional organisations and bodies representing health care professions should take immediate action in developing policies and guidelines on the identification and management of the problem in all health care settings/ such as accident and emergency departments, maternity units and general practices.

8   Organisations should disseminate such guidance widely in various formats including conferences and accessible materials such as short briefing papers, contact lists, best practice posters and reference booklets. Ongoing commitment to the implementation of guidelines and to staff training is required: regular audit of process outcomes and rates of identification may be useful in this respect.

9   Health care professionals should be aware of the importance of creating a safe and private environment for questioning and should develop a non-judgmental and supportive attitude towards domestic violence to both men and women. Men especially may find it hard to be believed.

10 All health professionals should obtain information about the local resources and initiatives available that would help an individual in the event of a disclosure of domestic violence. At a basic level this should include information on the local refuges, the police station and domestic violence unit, organisations that help children, organisations that offer legal advice and support and counselling groups.

11 Health professionals should liaise with organisations such as the Women's Aid Federation and other voluntary sector agencies who have taken a key role in supporting women who have experienced domestic violence, as part of a inter-agency approach. Inter-agency initiatives on domestic violence have a great deal to offer health care professionals, particularly in terms of training opportunities, information on support groups, resources and referral agencies and guidance on best policy and practice.

Education and training

12 All health professionals should be given basic information on the nature and prevalence of domestic violence including steps to be taken following disclosure of domestic violence.

13 Such education and training should be part of the undergraduate curriculum, specialist training curriculum and also part of structured training and continuing professional development programmes of the Royal Colleges and other professional bodies.

14 The major professional bodies representing the medical profession should develop education programmes and guidelines to include the careful documentation of all injuries of domestic violence and on producing medical evidence in written and oral forms for the courts.

Research

15 An extended and comprehensive research base is required on domestic violence in the UK and high quality research should be encouraged on the prevalence, identification and care of women experiencing domestic violence and also on the benefit (or otherwise) of screening in health care settings.

16 Further research into the short and long term health implications of domestic violence for both adults and children is required. The BMA Joan Dawkins Award has recently provided an award of £17,000 for research into the physical, psychological and social implications of domestic violence.

17 Detailed research on both the prevalence of male reported domestic violence and the circumstances in which it occurs is required.

18 Research is also required which looks specifically at medical practitioners' responses to domestic violence in black and ethnic minority families and in lesbian and gay relationships.

19 The relationship between disabilities and domestic violence requires further research, including those in community care and how to protect people who are 'cared' for in their homes. Services available to help women who experience domestic violence are seldom accessible to people with disabilities and little effort has been made to make them so. Disability groups have also shown little interest in domestic violence and in the accessibility of services for people with disabilities who suffer domestic violence.

20 The role of the medical profession in civil and criminal legal proceedings relating to domestic violence should be examined, and the findings of that research fed into education and training material for producing written and oral medical evidence for the courts.

21 A central database of domestic violence research and projects should be established for access by researchers, academics and agencies dealing with domestic violence, including the medical profession.

Appendix 1: Useful contacts

Agencies offering advice, information, refuge and practical support

Women's Aid National Office (refuge, legal advice, emotional support)
P O Box 391
Bristol
BS99 7WS
0117 944 4411 (office)
0345 023468 (24 hour national helpline)

London Women's Aid
P O Box 14041
London
E1 6NY
0171 392 2092 (24 hours)

Northern Ireland Women's Aid Federation
129 University Street
Belfast
BT7 1HP
01232 249041 or 01232 249358
01232 331818 (24 hour helpline)

Scottish Women's Aid
Norton Park
57 Albion Road
Edinburgh
EH7 5QY
0131 475 2372

Welsh Women's Aid

Cardiff

38-48 Crwys Road
Cardiff
CF2 4NN
01222 390874

Aberystwyth

4 Pound Place
Aberystwyth
SY23 1LX
01970 612748

Rhyl

2nd Floor
26b Wellington Road
Rhyl
Denbighshire
LL18 1BN
01745 334767
(These national groups can also refer to refuges catering for the needs of Asian, African, African Carribean, Chinese and Latin American Women)

Victim Support (National Office)

Cranmer House
39 Brixton Road
London
SW9 6DZ
0171 735 9050 (enquiries)

Victim Support Northern Ireland

Annsgate House
70/74 Ann Street
Belfast
BT1 4EH
01232 244039

Victim Support Scotland
14 Frederick Street
Edinburgh
EH2 2HB
0131 225 7779

Southall Black Sisters
52 Norwood Road
Southall
Middlesex
UB2 4DW
0181 571 9595

Jewish Women's Aid
PO Box 14270
London
N12 8WG
0800 591203 (freephone)
0171 486 0860 (office)

Refuge
2-8 Maltravers Street
London
WC2R 3EE
0171 395 7700 (office)
0990 995443 (24 hour crisis line)

Refuge for Women with Learning Difficulties
Beverley Lewis House
PO Box 7312
London
E15 4TS
0181 522 0675

Shelter National Campaign for the Homeless
0800 446441 (freephone)

Advice and legal advice

Rights of Women
52-54 Featherstone Street
London
EC1Y 8RT
0171 251 6577

Immigration Advisory Service
0171 378 9191

Lesbian and Gay Switchboard
0171 837 7324

Rape Crisis
P O Box 69
London
WC1X 9NJ
0171 837 1600

Local Solicitors
Especially those affiliated to the Solicitors Family Law Association, contact through local Yellow Pages directory or the Citizens Advice Bureau.

Agencies for parents and children

Childline
Freepost 1111
London
N1 0BR
0171 239 1000 (office)
0800 1111 (freephone)

Admin
Royal Mail Building
Studd Street
London
N1 0QW
0171 239 1000

Children's Legal Centre

University of Essex
Wivenhoe Park
Colchester
SYC0 43Q
01206 873820

National Society for the Protection of Cruelty to Children (NSPCC)

42 Curtain Road
London
EC2A 3NH
0171 825 2775

Other contacts

Alcoholics Anonymous

0171 352 3001 (national helpline)

Samaritans

0345 909090

Domestic Violence Intervention Project

0181 563 7983

Many local probation services are now involved in perpetrators' projects, contact
through local probation service offices.

References

Chapter 1

1   Bewley S, Friend J, Mezey G, eds. *Violence Against Women.* London: RCOG Press, 1997

2   World Medical Association. *Declaration on family violence. Adopted by the 48th General Assembly.* South Africa: October, 1996

3   Department of Health. *On the State of the Public Health: The Annual Report of the Chief Medical Officer of the Department of Health for the Year 1996.* London: HMSO, 1997

4   Department of Health. *The New NHS: White Paper.* Cm 3807 London: HMSO, 1997

5   Department of Health. *Our Healthier Nation: Green Paper.* London: HMSO,1998

6   Department of Health, Scottish Office. *Working together for a healthier Scotland.* Edinburgh: Scottish Office, 1998

7   See reference 5

8   See reference 6

9   See reference 4

10 Department of Health, Scottish Office. *Designed to Care — Renewing the NHS in Scotland.* London: The Stationery Office, 1997

Chapter 2

1   Home Affairs Committee. *Home Affairs Committee Report on Domestic Violence.* London: HMSO, 1993

2   Home Office and Welsh Office. *Domestic Violence: Don't Stand For It: Inter-Agency Co- ordination To Tackle Domestic Violence.* London: Home Office, 1995

3   Dobash RE and Dobash R. *Violence Against Wives: A Case Against The Patriarchy.* New York: Free Press, 1979

4   See reference 3

5   Mayhew P, Mirlees-Black C, Percy A. *The 1996 British Crime Survey England and Wales. Home Office Statistical Bulletin, Issue 19/96.* London: Home Office, 1996

6   Department of Health. *Our Healthier Nation: Green Paper.* London: HMSO,1998

7   See reference 5

8   Mirrlees-Black C. Estimating the extent of domestic violence: Findings from the 1992 British Crime Survey. In: *Home Office Research and Statistics Department Research Bulletin No. 37*. London: Home Office Research and Statistics Department, 1995

9   Johnson H, Sacco V. Researching Violence Against Women: Statistics Canada's National Survey. *Canadian Journal of Criminology* 1995; July: 281-304

10 Mooney J. *The Hidden Figure: Domestic Violence in North London*. Islington: Islington Council Police & Crime Prevention Unit, 1994

11 Stanko E, Crisp D, Hale C, Lucraft H. *Counting The Costs: Estimating The Impact of Domestic Violence in The London Borough of Hackney*. Children's Society/Hackney Safer Cities, 1997

12 Dominy N, Radford L. *Domestic Violence in Surrey: Developing An Effective Inter-Agency Response*. Surrey County Council/Roehampton Institute, 1996

13 Painter K. *Wife Rape, Marriage and the Law: Survey Report, Key Findings and Recommendations*. Manchester: University of Manchester, Faculty of Economic and Social Studies, 1991

14 Russell D. *Rape In Marriage*. Bloomington: Indiana University Press, 1982

15 See reference 5

16 Dobash R, Dobash RE. *Women, Violence and Social Change*. London: Routledge, 1992

17 Wilson M, Daly M. *Homicide*. New York: Aldine de Gruyter, 1988

18 See reference 9

19 Binney V, Harkell G, Nixon J. *Leaving Violent Men*. Bristol: Women's Aid Federation, 1988

20 See reference 8

21 See reference 10

22 Hester M, Radford L. *Domestic Violence and Child Contact Arrangements in England and Denmark*. Bristol: Policy Press, 1996

23 See reference 8

24 See reference 5

25 Edwards S. *Policing 'Domestic' Violence*. London: Sage, 1989

26 McGibbon A, Cooper L, Kelly L. *What Support?* Hammersmith & Fulham Council/Polytechnic of North London, 1988

27 Pahl J. *Private Violence and Public Policy*. London: Routledge, 1985

28 Grace S. *Policing Domestic Violence in the 1990s. Home Office Research Study No 139*. London: Home Office, 1995

29 Smith L. *Domestic Violence: A Review of the Literature. Home Office Research Study No. 107*. London: Home Office,1989

30 See reference 12

31 See reference 10

32 See reference 12

33 See reference 26

34 See reference 2

35 Smith M. Enhancing the Quality of Survey Data in Violence Against Women: A Feminist Approach. *Gender and Society* 1994;8(1):109-127

36 Flitcraft A. Learning From the Paradoxes of Domestic Violence. *Journal of the American Medical Association* 1997;277:1400-01

37 Richardson J, Feder G. Domestic violence: a hidden problem for general practice. *British Journal of General Practice* 1996:46:239-42

Chapter 3

1 Dobash RE, Dobash R, Cavanagh K, Lewis R. *Research Evaluation of Programmes for Violent Men*. Edinburgh: HMSO,1996

2 Jukes A. *Why Men Hate Women*. London: The Association Books, 1993

3 Schornstein S. *Domestic Violence And Health Care*. London: Sage, 1997

4 Domestic Abuse Intervention Project. Duluth: Minnesota

5 See reference 4

6 Yearnshire S. Analysis of Cohort. In: Bewley S, Friend J, Mezey G, eds. *Violence Against Women*. London: RCOG Press, 1997

7 Edleson J, Tolman R. *Intervention For Men Who Batter*. London: Sage, 1992

8 Hester M, Radford L. *Domestic Violence and Child Contact Arrangements in England and Denmark*. Bristol: Policy Press, 1996

9 Hester M, Pearson C, Radford L. *Domestic Violence: A National Survey of Family Court Welfare and Voluntary Sector Mediation Practice*. Bristol: Policy Press, 1997

10 Browne A. *When Battered Women Kill*. New York: Free Press, 1987

11 Glass D. *All My Fault: Why Women Don't Leave Abusive Men*. London: Virago, 1997

12 See reference 10

13   See reference 8

14   Walker LE. *The Battered Woman.* New York: Harpers and Row, 1979

15   Biennia V, Harked G, Nikon J. *Leaving Violent Men.* Bristol: Women's Aid Federation, 1981

16   Hoof L. *Battered Women As Survivors.* London: Routledge, 1990

17   Pahl J. *Private Violence and Public Policy.* London: Routledge, 1985

18   McWilliams M, McKiernan J. *Bringing It Out In The Open: Domestic Violence in Northern Ireland.* Belfast: HMSO, 1993

19   See reference 17

20   See reference 17

21   Mooney J. *The Hidden Figure: Domestic Violence in North London.* Islington: Islington Council Police & Crime Prevention Unit, 1994

22   Ferrante A, Morgan F, Indermaur D, Harding R. *Measuring The Extent of Domestic Violence.* Sydney: Hawkins Press, 1996

23   Mirrlees-Black C. Estimating the extent of domestic violence: findings from the 1992 British Crime Survey. In: *Home Office Research and Statistics Department Research Bulletin No.37.* London: Home Office Research and Statistics Department, 1995

24   Pahl J. *Money & Marriage.* Basingstoke: Macmillan, 1989

25   Rathbone E. *The Disinherited Family.* Birkenhead: Wilmer Bros & Co, 1924

26   Graham H. *Hardship and Health in Women's Lives.* Hemel Hempstead: Harvester/Wheatsheaf, 1993

27   Department of Health. *Our Healthier Nation: Green Paper.* London: HMSO,1998

28   Women's Local Authority Network. *Progressing The Agenda: Further Local Authority Initiatives to Counter Violence Against Women.* Manchester: Women's Local Authority Network, 1996

29   British Medical Association. *Meeting the needs of doctors with disabilities.* London: BMA, 1997

30   British Medical Association. *Discrimination on the grounds of sexual orientation.* London: BMA, in print

31   Bhatti-Sinclair K. Asian Women and Violence From Male Partners. In: Lupton C, Gillespie T, eds. *Working With Violence.* London: Macmillan/British Association of Social Workers, 1994

32   Mama A. *The Hidden Struggle: Statutory and Voluntary Sector Responses to Violence Against Black Women in the Home.* London: London Race and Housing Unit, 1989

33   Southall Black Sisters. Domestic Violence and Immigration Law: An Urgent Need For Reform. In: *Home Affairs Select Committee Report on Domestic Violence. Volume 2:Appendix 9.* London: HMSO, 1993

34 Hester M, Radford L. *Domestic Violence and Child Contact Arrangements in England and Denmark*. Bristol: Policy Press, 1996

35 See reference 32

36 See reference 27

37 Renzetti C. *Violent Betrayal: Partner Abuse in Lesbian Relationships*. London: Sage, 1992

38 Hart B. Lesbian Battering: An Examination. In: Lobel K, ed. *Naming the Violence: Speaking Out About Lesbian Battering*. Washington: Seal Press, 1986

39 See reference 28

40 Letellier P. Twin Epidemics: Domestic Violence and HIV Infection Among Gay and Bisexual Men. In: Renzetti C, Miley C, eds. *Violence in Gay and Lesbian Domestic Partnerships*. New York: Harrington Park, 1996

41 Chenoweth L. Violence and Women With Disabilities: Silence and Paradox. In: Cook S, Bessant J, eds. *Women's Encounters With Violence: Australian Experiences*. California: Sage, 1997

42 Mullender A. *Re-Thinking Domestic Violence: The Social Work and Probation Response*. London: Routledge, 1996

43 McCarthy M. Sexual Experiences and Sexual Abuse of Women With Learning Disabilities. In: Hester M, Kelly L, Radford J, eds. *Women, Violence and Male Power*. Milton Keynes: Open University Press, 1996

44 Cosgrove K, Macleod J. *We're No Exception: Male Violence Against Women With Disability*. Glasgow: Zero Tolerance Campaign, 1995

45 Stark E, Flitcraft A. *Women At Risk: Domestic Violence and Women's Health*. London: Sage, 1996

46 Dobash RE, Dobash R. *Violence Against Wives: A Case Against The Patriarchy*. New York: Free Press, 1979

47 Mayhew P, Mirlees-Black C, Percy A. *The 1996 British Crime Survey England and Wales, Home Office Statistical Bulletin, Issue 19/96*. London: Home Office, 1996

48 See reference 45

49 See reference 45

50 Mullender A, Morley R, eds. *Children Living With Domestic Violence: Putting Men's Abuse of Women on the Child Care Agenda*. London: Whiting and Birch, 1994

51 See reference 42

52 See reference 50

53 Mezey G. Perpetrators of Domestic Violence. In: Bewley S, Friend J, Mezey G, eds. *Violence Against Women* London: RCOG Press, 1997

54 Crowell N, Burgess A, eds. *Understanding Violence Against Women*. Washington DC: National Academy Press, 1996

55 George M. Violence Against Men. In: *Home Affairs Select Committee Report on Domestic Violence*. London: HMSO, 1993

56 Thomas D. *Not Guilty: In Defence of The Modern Man*. London: Weidenfeld & Nicolson, 1994

57 Mirlees-Black C. Personal communication, 1998

58 Home Office. *Criminal Statistics*. London: Home Office Research and Statistics Department, 1992

59 Wilson M, Johnson H, Daly M. Lethal and Non-Lethal Violence Against Wives. *Canadian Journal Of Criminology* 1995; July

60 Radford L. Pleading For Time: Justice For Battered Women Who Kill. In:Birch H, ed. *Moving Targets*. London: Virago, 1993

61 Straus M, Gelles R, Steinmetz S. *Behind Closed Doors: Violence in The American Family*. New York: Doubleday/Anchor, 1980

62 See reference 42

63 Dobash RE, Dobash R. *Women, Violence and Social Change*. London: Routledge, 1992

64 Gelles R, Pedrick-Cornell C. *Intimate Violence in Families*. London: Sage, 1990

65 Families Need Fathers. In: *House of Commons Home Affairs Select Committee Report on Domestic Violence*. London: HMSO, 1993

66 See reference 42

67 Ball M. *Funding Refuge Services: A Study of Refuge Support Services For Women and Children Experiencing Domestic Violence*. London: HMSO, 1994

Chapter 4

1 Richardson J, Feder G. Domestic violence: a hidden problem for general practice. *British Journal of General Practice* 1996;46:239-42

2 Mullender A, Morley R. *Children Living With Domestic Violence: Putting men's abuse of women on the child care agenda*. London: Whiting and Birch, 1994

3 Stanko E, Crisp D, Hale C, Lucraft H. *Counting the Costs: Estimating the Impact of Domestic Violence in the London Borough of Hackney*. Crime Concern, 1997

4 Stark E, Flitcraft AH. Spouse abuse. In: Rosenberg M, Mercy J, eds. *Violence in America: a public health approach*. New York: Oxford University Press, 1991

5 Gazmararian JA, Lazorick S, Spitz AM, Ballard TJ, Saltzman LE, Marks JS. Prevalence of domestic violence against pregnant women. *Journal of the American Medical Association* 1996;275:1915-20

6 Bullock L, McFarlane J, Bateman LH, Miller V. The prevalence and characteristics of battered women in a primary care setting. *Nurse Practitioner* 1989;14:47-56

7 Stewart DE. Incidence of postpartum abuse in women with a history of abuse during pregnancy. *Canadian Medical Association Journal* 1994;151:1601-4

8 Stark E, Flitcraft A, Frazier W. Medicine and patriarchal violence: the social construction of a private event. *International Journal of Health Services* 1979;9:461-93

9 Bullock LF, McFarlane J. The birth-weight/battering connection. *American Journal of Nursing* 1989;89:1153-55

10 Cascy M. *Domestic Violence Against Women: The Women's Perspective.* Dublin: Social Psychology Research Unit, UCD, 1989

11 McWilliams M, McKiernan J. *Bringing It Out In The Open: Domestic Violence in Northern Ireland.* Belfast: HMSO, 1993

12 See reference 3

13 See reference 11

14 Dominy N, Radford L. *Domestic Violence in Surrey: Towards an Effective Inter-Agency Approach.* Surrey County Council/Roehampton Institute, 1996

15 Bang L. Rape victims - assaults, injuries and treatment at a medical rape trauma service at Oslo Emergency Hospital. *Scandinavian Journal of Primary Health Care* 1993;11:15- 20

16 Whatley MA. For better or worse: The case of marital rape. *Violence and Victims* 1993;8:29-39

17 Hampton HL. Care of the woman who has been raped. *New England Journal of Medicine* 1995;322:234-7

18 Womens Aid Federation of England. *Womens Education Project. Breaking through: Women surviving male violence.* Bristol: WAFE, 1989

19 Walker L. The Battered Woman. New York: Harper and Row, 1979

20 Schornstein S. *Domestic Violence and Health Care: What every professional needs to know.* London: Sage, 1997

21 Richardson J. Women and domestic violence. CML-Psychiatry 1996;7:87-91

22 Jacobson A, Richardson B. Assault experiences of 100 psychiatric in-patients: Evidence for the need for routine inquiry. *American Journal of Psychiatry* 1987;144: 908-13

23 See reference 21

24 See reference 14

25 Hoff L. *Battered Women As Survivors*. London: Routledge, 1990

26 Kirkwood C. *Leaving Abusive Partners*. London: Sage, 1993

27 Bewley S, Friend J, Mezey G, eds. *Violence Against Women*. London: RCOG Press, 1997

28 See reference 25

29 See reference 14

30 See reference 4

31 Plichta S. The effects of woman abuse on health care utilisation and health status:a literature review. *Women's Health Issues* 1992;2:154-63

32 Stark E, Flitcraft A. *Women At Risk: Domestic Violence and Women's Health*. London: Sage, 1996

33 Hanmer J. Women and Policing in Britain. In Hanmer J, Radford J, Stanko E, eds. *Women, Policing and Male Violence*. London: Routledge, 1989

34 Jaffe P, Wolfe D, Wilson S. *Children of Battered Women*. London: Sage, 1990

35 Silvern L, Karyl J, Landis T. Individualised Psychotherapy for Traumatised Children of Abused Women. In: Pelad E, Jaffe P, Edleson J, eds. *Ending The Cycle of Violence: Community Responses to Children of Battered Women*. London: Sage, 1995

36 Hester M, Radford L. *Domestic Violence and Child Contact Arrangements in England and Denmark*. Bristol: Policy Press, 1996

37 Saunders A. *It Hurts Me Too: Children's Experiences of Domestic Violence and Refuge Life*. London: Women's Aid Federation England/National Institute for Social Work/ChildLine, 1995

38 See reference 36

39 Pahl J. *Private Violence and Public Policy*. London: Routledge, 1985

40 See reference 36

41 Binney V, Harkell G, Nixon J. *Leaving Violent Men*. Bristol: Women's Aid Federation, 1981

42 Bowker L, Arbitell M, McFerron J. On the Relationship Between Wife Beating and Child Abuse. In Yllo K, Bograd M, eds. *Feminist Perspectives on Wife Abuse*. London: Sage, 1988

43 See reference 32

44 Brandon M, Lewis A. Significant Harm and the Children's Experiences of Domestic Violence. *Child and Family Social Work* 1996;1(1):33-42

45 Farmer E, Owen M. *Child Protection Practice: Private Risks and Public Remedies*, London: HMSO, 1995

46 Hester M, Pearson C. *Preventing Child Abuse - Monitoring Domestic Violence*. Bristol: Policy Press, 1998 (forthcoming)

47 NSPCC. Press Release. May 1998

48 NCH Action For Children. *The Hidden Victims: Children and Domestic Violence*. London: NCH Action For Children, 1994

49 See reference 36

50 See reference 41

51 See reference 2

52 Mullender A. *Re-Thinking Domestic Violence: The Social Work and Probation Response*, London: Routledge, 1996

53 Hester M, Malos E, Hague G. *Domestic Violence and Children - A Reader*. London: Barnados/Department of Health, 1998 (forthcoming)

54 See reference 2

55 See reference 48

56 See reference 46

57 See reference 33

58 See reference 34

59 See reference 34

60 See reference 34

61 See reference 36

62 See reference 36

63 See reference 36

64 See reference 36

65 See reference 54

66 Crowell N, Burgess A, eds. *Understanding Violence Against Women*. Washington DC: National Academy Press, 1996

67 See reference 3

68 See reference 3

69 See reference 3

70 See reference 10

71 See reference 14

72 See reference 3

Chapter 5

1 Stark E, Flitcraft AH. Spouse abuse. In: Rosenberg M, Mercy J, eds. *Violence in America: a public health approach.* New York: Oxford University Press, 1991

2 Ferris EL. Canadian family Doctors' and General Practitioners' Perceptions of their Effectiveness in Identifying and Treating Wife Abuse. *Medical Care* 1994;32:1163- 72

3 Sugg NK, Inui T. Primary care doctors' response to domestic violence. Opening Pandora's box. *Journal of the American Medical Association* 1992;267:3157-60

4 Brown JB, Lent B, Sas G. Identifying and treating wife abuse. *Journal of Family Practice* 1993;36:185-91

5 Warshaw C. Domestic violence: challenges to medical practice. *Journal of Women's Health* 1993;2:73-80

6 Warshaw C. Limitations of the medical model in the care of battered women. *Gender and Society* 1989;3:506-517

7 Pahl J. The general practitioner and the problems of battered women. *Journal Medical Ethics* 1979;5:117-23

8 Hopayian K, Horrocks G, Garner P, Levitt A. Battered women presenting in general practice. *Journal of the Royal College of General Practitioners* 1983;33:506-7

9 Dobash RE, Dobash RP. *Violence against wives. A Case against the Patriarchy.* London; Open Books, 1979

10 Binney V, Harkell G, Nixon J. *Leaving violent men. A study of refuges and housing for battered women.* Bristol: Women's Aid Federation England, 1981

11 McGibbon AC, Fulham Council Community Police Committee. *Domestic Violence Project.* The Polytechnic of North London, 1989

12 Mooney J. *The Hidden Figure: domestic violence in North London.* London: Islington Council, 1993

13 Dominy N, Radford L. *Domestic Violence in Surrey: Developing an effective inter-agency response.* Surrey County Council/Roehampton Institute, 1996

14 Mazza D, Dennerstein L, Ryan V. Physical, sexual and emotional violence against women: a general practice-based prevalence study. *Medical Journal of Australia* 1996;164:14- 17

15 Mezey G, King M, McClintock T. Victims of violence and the GP. *British Journal of General Practice* 1998:48:906-908

16 See reference 15

17 Friedman LS, Samet JH, Roberts MS, Hudlin M, Hans P. Inquiry about victimization experiences. A survey of patient preferences and doctor practices. *Archives of Internal Medicine* 1992;152:1186-90

18 McWilliams M, McKiernan J. *Bringing it out in the open: domestic violence in Northern Ireland.* Belfast: HMSO, 1993

19 Mezey G, King M, MacClintock T. Victims of violence and the general practitioner. *British Journal of General Practice* 1998;48:906-8

20 Anonymous. American Medical Association Diagnostic and Treatment Guidelines on Domestic Violence. *Archives of Family Medicine* 1992;1:39-47

21 Heath I. *Domestic violence: the general practitioners role. Royal College of General Practitioners Members Reference Book 1992.* London: Sabrecrown, 1992

22 Centers for Disease Control. Education about adult domestic violence in US and Canadian medical schools 1987-88. *Journal of the American Medical Association* 1989;261:972-8

23 Alpert EJ, Tonkin AE, Seeherman AM, Holtz HA. *Family violence and the medical school curriculum. Paper presented at the Annual Meeting of the Association of American Medical Colleges.* Boston, MA, October 1994

24 Abbott P, Williamson E. *Women, health and domestic violence.* Paper presented at the BSA Medical Conference, 1997

25 West Glasgow Hospitals University NHS Trust Accident and Emergency Department. *Protocol on Domestic Violence: Open Learning Pack.* Glasgow, 1995

26 McLeer SV, Anwar RAH, Herman S, Maculing K. Education is not enough: a systems failure in protecting battered women. *Annals of Emergency Medicine* 1989;18:651-3

27 Alpert EJ, Cohen S, eds. Educating the Nation's Physicians about Family Violence and Abuse. *Academic Medicine* 1997;72(1) Jan Supplement:S1-115

28 Warshaw C. Intimate partner abuse: developing a framework for change in medical education. *Academic Medicine* 1997;72(1) Jan Supplement:S26-S37

29 See reference 28

30 Short LM, Cotton D, Hodgson CS. Evaluation of the module on domestic violence at the UCLA school of medicine. *Academic Medicine* 1997;72(1) Jan Supplement S72-92

31 Saunders DG, Kindy P. Predictors of doctors responses to woman abuse; the role of gender, background and brief training. *Journal of General Internal Medicine* 1993;8:606-9

32 Varvaro FF, Gesmond S. Emergency department physician house staff response to training on domestic violence. *Journal of Emergency Nursing* 1997:23:17-22

Chapter 6

1   McFarlane J, Greenberg L, Weltge A, Watson M. Identification of abuse in emergency departments: Effectiveness of a two-question screening tool. *Journal of Emergency Nursing* 1995;21:391-4

2   Feldhaus KM, Koziol-McLain J, Amsbury HL, Norton IM, Lowenstein SR, Abbott JT. Accuracy of three brief screening questions for detecting partner violence in the emergency department. *Journal of the American Medical Association* 1997;277:1357-61

3   Anonymous. American Medical Association Diagnostic and Treatment Guidelines on Domestic Violence. *Archives of Family Medicine* 1992;1:39-47

4   Campbell JC. Nursing assessment for risk of homicide with battered women. *Advances in Nursing Science* 1986;8:36-51

5   Mama A. *The hidden struggle: statutory and voluntary sector responses to violence against black women in the home.* London: London Race and Housing Unit, 1989

6   Schuler SR, Hashemi SM, Riley A, Akhter S. Credit programs, patriarchy and men's violence against women in rural Bangladesh. *Social Science and Medicine* 1996; 43: 1729-42

7   Heath I. *Domestic violence: the general practitioner's role. Royal College of General Practitioners Members Reference Book 1992.* London: Sabrecrown, 1992

8   Alpert EJ. Violence in intimate relationships and the practising internist: new 'disease' or new agenda? *Annals of Internal Medicine* 1995;123:774-81

9   Pahl J. Health professionals and violence against women. In: Kingston P, Penhale B, eds. *Family violence and the caring professions.* London: Macmillan, 1995

10 See reference 7

11 See reference 8

12 Sheridan DJ, Taylor WK. Developing hospital-based domestic violence programs, protocols, policies and procedures. *AWHONNS Clinical Issues in Perinatal and Womens Health Nursing* 1993;4:471-82

13 Bewley S, Friend J, Mezey G, eds. *Violence Against Women.* London: RCOG Press, 1997

14 General Medical Council. *Duties of a Doctor: Confidentiality.* GMC 1995

15 See reference 14

16 BMA, GMSC, HEA, Brook Advisory Centres, FPA, RCGP. *Confidentiality and People Under 16.* 1994

Chapter 7

1　Davison J. Domestic Violence: the nursing response. *Professional Nurse* 1997;12(9):617

2　Dobash RP, Dobash RE. *Women, Violence and Social Change*. London, Routledge, 1992

3　Stevens KLH. The role of the accident and emergency department. In: Bewley S, Friend J, Mezey G, eds. *Violence Against Women*. London: RCOG Press, 1997

4　See reference 3

5　Bergman B, Brismar B. Battered Wives — measured by the social and medical services. *Postgraduate Medical Journal* 1990:66; 28-33

6　See reference 3

7　Norton LB, Peipert JF, Zierler S, Lima B, Hume L. Battering in pregnancy: an assessment of two screening methods. *Obstetrics and Gynaecology* 1995:85;321-5

8　McLeer SV, Anwar RA, Herman S, Maculing K. Education is not enough: a systems failure in protecting battered women. *Annals of Emergency Medicine* 1989:18;651-3

9　Helton A, McFarlane J, Anderson E. Prevention of battering during pregnancy; focus on behavioural change. *Public Health Nursing* 1987:4;166-74

10　Bokunewicz B, Copel LC. Attitudes of emergency nurses before and after a 60-minute educational presentation on partner abuse. *Journal of Emergency Nursing*. 1992:18;24-27

11　See reference 3

12　British Association of Accident and Emergency Medicine. *Domestic Violence: Recognition and Management in Accident and Emergency*. London: Royal College of Surgeons, 1994

13　Hillard PA. Physical abuse in pregnancy. *Obstetrics and Gynaecology* 1985:66;185-190

14　Bohn DK. Domestic Violence and Pregnancy: Implications for practice. *Journal of Nurse Midwifery* 1990:35;86-98

15　Gielen AC, O'Campo PJ, Faden RR, Kass NE, Xue X. Interpersonal conflict and physical violence during the childbearing year. *Social Science Medicine* 1994;39:781-7

16　Berenson AB, Wiemann CM, Wilkinson GS, Jones WA, Anderson GD. Perinatal morbidity associated with violence experienced by pregnant women. *American Journal of Obstetrics and Gynaecology* 1994;170:1760-9

17　Bewley S, Friend J, Mezey G (eds.). *Violence Against Women*. London, RCOG Press, 1997

18　Parsons LH, Zaccaro D, Wells B, Stovall TG. Methods of and attitude towards screening obstetrics and gynaecology patients for domestic violence. *American Journal of Obstetrics and Gynaecology* 1995;173(2):381-6

19   McFarlane J. Battering during pregnancy: tip of an iceberg revealed. *Women's Health* 1989:15;69-84

20   See reference 7

21   See reference 17

22   Roberts GL, Lawrence J M, O'Toole BI, Raphael B. Domestic Violence in the Emergency Department: I Two case-control studies of victims. *General Hospital Psychiatry* 1997:19;5-11

23   Herman JL. Histories of violence in an outpatient population: an exploratory study. *American Journal of Orthopsychiatry* 1986;56(1);137-141

24   See reference 22

25   See reference 22

26   Ratner PA. Indicators of exposure to wife abuse. *Canadian Journal of Nursing Research.* 1995;27(1):31-46

27   See reference 1

28   Langley H. The health professionals: an overview. In: Bewley S, Friend J, Mezey, eds. *Violence Against Women.* London, RCOG Press, 1997

29   Mezey G, King M, MacClintock T. Victims of Violence and the General Practitioner. *British Journal of General Practice* 1998:48:906-908

30   See reference 14

31   See reference 16

32   Royal College of Midwives. *Domestic Abuse in Pregnancy. Position Paper 19.* London: RCM, 1997

33   See reference 7

34   MacFarlane J, Parker B, Soeken K, Bullock L. Assessing for abuse during pregnancy. *Journal of the American Medical Association* 1992;267:3176-8

35   Bewley CA, Gibbs A. Violence in pregnancy. *Midwifery* 1991;7:107-12

Chapter 8

1   Hague G, Malos E, Dear W. *Multi-Agency Work and Domestic Violence: A National Study of Inter-Agency Initiatives.* Bristol : Policy Press, 1997

2   Dominy N, Radford L. *Domestic Violence in Surrey: Towards an Effective Inter-Agency Response.* Surrey County Council/Roehampton Institute, 1996

3   McCartney, S. *Report on Greater Glasgow Health Board's Health Gain Commissioning Team on Domestic Violence.* Glasgow: Greater Glasgow Health Board, Department of Public Health, 1997

4 Harwin N, Malos E, Hague G, eds. *Inter-Agency Responses to Domestic Violence*. London: Whiting and Birch, 1998

5 Hague G, Malos E, Dear W. *Against Domestic Violence: Inter-agency Initiatives. Working Paper 127.* Bristol: SAUS Publications, 1995

6 Reid S, Glasser M. Primary Care Doctors' Recognition of and Attitudes Toward Domestic Violence. *Academic Medicine* 1997; 72;1:51-53

7 Home Office and Welsh Office. *Domestic Violence: Don't Stand For It: Inter-Agency Co-ordination To Tackle Domestic Violence.* London: Home Office, 1995

8 Department of Health. *Our Healthier Nation: Green Paper.* HMSO; London, 1998

9 Edwards S. *Policing Domestic Violence.* London: Sage, 1989

10 See reference 9

11 Mama A. *The Hidden Struggle.* London: London Race and Housing Research Unit, 1989

12 Southall Black Sisters. *Memorandum to the Home Affairs Committee Third Report: Domestic Violence, Vol II Memoranda of Evidence, Minutes of Evidence and Appendices, Appendix 9.* London: HMSO, 1993

13 Home Office. *Guidance to Chief Officers of Police in dealing with Domestic Violence. Circular 60/1990.* London: Home Office, July 1990

14 See reference 2

15 Butler E. *Domestic Violence: Surrey Inter-Agency Guidelines and Information Pack.* Godalming: Surrey Domestic Violence Project, 1998

16 Grace S. *Policing Domestic Violence in the 1990s. Home Office Research Study 139.* London: HMSO, 1995

17 HM Inspectorate of Constabulary. *Hitting Home - A report on the Police Response to Domestic Violence.* Scotland: HM Inspectorate of Constabulary, 1997

18 Department of Health. *Working Together LAC (91)17.* London: Department of Health, 1991

19 Surrey Area Child Protection Committee. *Manual of Child Protection Procedures.* Guildford: Surrey Social Services, 1996

20 Mullender A, Morley R, eds. *Children Living Through Domestic Violence: Putting Men's Abuse of Women on the Child Care Agenda.* London: Whiting and Birch, 1994

21 Malos E, Hague G. *Domestic Violence and Housing.* Bristol: Women's Aid Federation England/University of Bristol, 1993

22 Edleson J, Tolman R. *Intervention For Men Who Batter.* London: Sage, 1992

23 Burton S, Regan L, Kelly L. *Supporting Women and Challenging Men: Lessons From The Domestic Violence Intervention Project.* Bristol: Policy Press, 1998

24 Dobash RE, Dobash R, Cavanagh K, Lewis R. *Research Evaluation of Programmes For Violent Men.* Edinburgh: HMSO, 1996

Chapter 9

1   Mayhew P, Aye Maung N, Mirrlees-Black C. *The British Crime Survey of England and Wales 1992. Home Office Research Study 132.* London: HMSO, 1993

2   Mayhew P, Mirrlees-Black C, Percy A. *The 1996 British Crime Survey England and Wales, Home Office Statistical Bulletin. Issue 19/96.* London: Home Office, 1996

3   Bewley S, Friend J, Mezey G, eds. *Violence Against Women.* London: RCOG Press, 1997

4   George M. Violence Against Men. In: *Home Affairs Select Committee Report on Domestic Violence.* London: HMSO, 1993

5   Department of Health. *On the State of the Public Health: The Annual Report of the Chief Medical Officer of the Department of Health for the Year 1996.* London: HMSO, 1997

6   Department of Health. *Our Healthier Nation: Green Paper.* London: HMSO, 1998

7   Department of Health, Scottish Office. *Working together for a healthier Scotland.* Edinburgh: Scottish Office, 1998

8   Department of Health. *The New NHS: White Paper.* Cm 3807 London: HMSO, 1997

9   Department of Health, Scottish Office. *Designed to Care - Renewing the NHS in Scotland.* London: The Stationery Office, 1997

10 See reference 7

11 See reference 6

12 Stevens, KLH. The role of the accident and emergency department. In: Bewley S, Friend J, Mezey G, eds. *Violence Against Women.* London: RCOG Press, 1997

13 Bewley S, Friend J, Mezey G, eds. *Violence Against Women.* London: RCOG Press, 1997

Index